ALLE ZEIT WACH 1842

A. Weissman M. Clot J. Grellet

Double Contrast Examination of the Colon

Principles and Practice

With a Foreword by Igor Laufer

With 172 Figures

Springer-Verlag
Berlin Heidelberg New York Tokyo

ALAIN WEISSMAN, MD
JACQUES GRELLET, MD, Professor of Radiology
Service Central de Radiologie
Groupe Hospitalier Pitie-Salpétriere
83, Boulevard de l'Hôpital
F-75651 Paris Cedex 13

MICHEL CLOT, MD
Clinique du Castel
24, Rue Jean Jaures
F-95600 Eaubonne

Translator
RICHARD T. CHAMBERS
9 bis, Rue de la Grette
F-25000 Besançon

Title of the original French edition
La mucographie colique by A. Weissman, M. Clot, J. Grellet
© Edition Pep Paris, 1979

ISBN-13: 978-3-642-70397-3 e-ISBN-13: 978-3-642-70395-9
DOI: 10.1007/978-3-642-70395-9

Library of Congress Cataloging in Publication Data. Weissman, Alain, 1946- . Double contrast examination of the colon. Translation of: La mucographie colique. Includes bibliographies and index. 1. Colon (Anatomy)-Radiography. 2. Radiography, Double-contrast. 3. Colon (Anatomy)-Diseases-Diagnosis. I. Clot, Michel, 1943- . II. Grellet, Jacques, 1931- . III. Title. RC804.R6W4513 1985 616.3'4 85-9727

Softcover reprint of the hardcover 1st edition 1985

Printing and bookbinding: Appl, Wemding
2121/3130-543210

Foreword

It is a great pleasure for me to introduce and to recommend this much needed text on double contrast examination of the colon. It is aimed both at clinicians who request X-ray examinations of the colon and at radiologists who must perform and interpret these studies.

Over the past decade there has been renewed interest in X-ray examination of the colon despite the tremendous advances in endoscopy and imaging technology. This renewed interest is evidenced by the proliferation of new books on radiology of the colon. However, previous discussions of double contrast examination have concentrated primarily on the technique with too little attention to the understanding and interpretation of the radiologic images.

This volume is unique in its emphasis on the basics of image formation and interpretation. It emphasizes the importance of the anteroposterior relationships of the colon in determining the distribution of barium and air. It also recognizes the influence of location on the radiologic appearance of the lesion.

The authors demonstrate a profound understanding of the principles of double contrast diagnosis as applied to the colon. They also have a good grasp of the gross pathologic changes underlying the radiologic images. The material is presented in a logical and analytical method which should be particularly useful to the beginner in this field. There are many helpful diagrams and the radiographic illustrations are of excellent quality.

I have no doubt that this volume will be of great benefit to all trainees in radiology and to practicing radiologists starting to do or wanting to improve and refine the quality of their double contrast examinations. It will also be a great help to many clinicians who may have been baffled by the mysteries of double contrast colonic radiography.

Radiographic examination of the colon has two components. In the first place, high quality radiographs must be obtained. This can be likened to the painting of a portrait. Secondly, the painter must be able to translate from the language of the radiograph to the language of gross pathology. One of the great virtues of this small volume is that it pays proper respect to both components of the examination.

In this era of explosive developments in technology and of the ever increasing cost of medical care, we owe a great debt of gratitude to Drs. Weissman, Clot, and Grellet for reminding us that the double contrast enema remains a most sensitive technique and is capable of exquisite beauty and life-saving diagnostic accuracy.

IGOR LAUFER, M.D.

Contents

1 Double Contrast Enema: Technical Aspects

The technique described here is one we have perfected and used for 10 years. Since our earlier work it has undergone certain changes, resulting in a more simplified procedure. In its broad outline, it is the same as that described by Welin [15]. Other methods have been successfully used by different authors [2, 4, 5, 7, 8]. They are based on the same principles: *the colonic mucosa (clean and cleared of secretions) is coated with a fine layer of adherent barium and the colon is distended by air insufflation.* Three conditions are essential for carrying out this procedure: (1) thorough preparation of the colon, (2) use of dense and adherent barium, (3) a full understanding of the technique, which is based on the use of a small quantity of barium "guided" to the cecum by changing the patient's position and gradually increasing the amount of air insufflated.

1.1 Preparation of the Patient

1.1.1 Objectives

This chapter will enable:

1. The practitioner (a) to point out to the radiologist the clinical means which will best allow the radiologist to adapt the preparation to the patient's condition. (b) to stress the importance to the patient of completely following the preparation instructions which must result in emptying the colon (purgatives, low-residue diet, etc.).

2. The specialist (a) to plan efficiently the preparation of the patient taking into account the clinical findings provided by the practitioner and the available technical means. (b) to learn the preparation technique, which is an indispensable prerequisite. It is impossible to carry out a diagnostic examination to a high standard in a poorly prepared patient.

It is the responsibility of the specialist who is to make the examination to choose the most suitable and most efficient preparation. This should take into account the conditions in which the examination is to be performed and the patient's symptoms and physiologic condition. The best preparations are those which comprise three parts: low-residue diet, laxatives, and cleansing enemas. Practical considerations are also important: shortest preparation time possible, ease of carrying it out, and good tolerance.

Poor results for the preparations in normal use seem to be due to: (1) the unrealistic nature of instructions, which are too complicated (prolonged diet for working patients, poor technique for enemas carried out at home by the patients themselves), (2) nonadherence to instructions (hospital staff inefficiency, lack of communication between practitioner and receptionist or patient), and (3) incomplete instructions.

1.1.2 Procedure

Preparation of ambulatory and bedridden patients (hospitalized) may be different, the latter being more difficult.

1.1.2.1 Ambulatory Patients

For adults, we use a preparation combining: (1) a low-residue diet and plenty of liquids during the 18–24 h prior to the examination (Tables 1.1, 1.2); (2) laxatives (magnesium sulfate, 24 g; and 2 × 4 tablets of Peristaltine[1]); timing for these prescriptions depends on whether the examination is carried out in the morning (Table 1.1) or afternoon (Table 1.2), and (3) atropine sulfate (1 mg) is taken orally ½ h prior to the examination. Glucagon (0.5 mg) may be given intravenously for patients with glaucoma or prostate complaints. Laxative doses are reduced for children.

This preparation was the object of a retrospective study of 100 cases. Results are shown in Table 1.3, from which it appears that excellent results were obtained in only 64% of the cases. In view of this, we now feel it is preferable, when possible, to add a cleansing enema the night before the examination or, in the morning, at the patient's home or in the Radiology Department. This latter is ideal, but greatly increases the examination time (2–3 h).

Two points seem to be essential for obtaining good results:

1. The need to explain the instructions to the patient personally and to stress the importance of following them completely. It is also necessary to explain the practical implications, such as buying medication and prescribed food in advance; probable frequent bowel movements, which may be a problem in certain cases; and making the appointment accordingly.

2. The need to adapt the preparation for particular cases: (a) severe diarrhea where organic colitis is suspected (or more than three bowel movements/day): lower laxative doses either immediately or after the first dose if followed by a rapid increase in fecal movement; (b) severe constipation: diet and laxatives for 2 days, change of laxative in favor of one which usually works for the patient or, if necessary, use of cleansing enemas; (c) dehydration: a preparation which combines laxatives and a diet of low-hydrated foods causes dehydration. This should be compensated for by drinking fluids (at least 2 liters). If such a diet affects the patient's general health, cleansing enemas can replace or accompany the oral preparation.

---

1 Anthraquinone obtained from *Rhamnus purshiana*, 0.100 g/tablet; Ciba Laboratories, 556 Maurice Avenue, Summit, NJ 07901, USA

Table 1.1. Preparation for a morning double contrast enema (preparation A)

N.B. These instructions must be followed exactly; the quality of the examination depends on it	
1. Preceding day	Before breakfast (8:00 AM): take one 8-g packet of magnesium sulfate dissolved in a glass of sugar water and four Peristaltine tablets Breakfast: coffee (no milk), sugar, dry toast (2), one hard-boiled egg, no bread 9:00-12:00 AM: no food; fluids as desired Lunch: fish or chicken, slice of cheese, dry toast (2-4), fruit jelly or honey, beverages as desired (sugared or not); no fatty foods, vegetables, fruit, rice, or bread Dinner (7:00 PM): clear broth (no vegetable soup), fruit jelly or honey with dry toast 8:30 PM: two 8-g packets of magnesium sulfate dissolved in a glass of sugar water and four Peristaltine tablets Drink plenty of fluids: at least 2 liters during the day
2. The day of the examination	Coffee without milk is permitted. No bread Take two atropine capsules ½ h before the examination

Table 1.2. Preparation for an afternoon double contrast enema (preparation B)

N.B. These instructions must be followed exactly; the quality of the examination depends on it	
1. Preceding day	Before breakfast (8:00 AM): take two 8-g packet of magnesium sulfate dissolved in a glass of sugar water and four Peristaltine tablets Breakfast: coffee (no milk), sugar, dry toast (2), one hard-boiled egg, no bread 9:00-12:00 AM: no food; fluids as desired Lunch: one hard-boiled egg or slice of ham, fish or chicken, slice of cheese, dry toast (2-4) with fruit jelly or honey. Beverages as desired (sugared or not). No fatty foods, vegetables, fruit, rice, or bread Dinner (7:00 PM): clear broth, one hard-boiled egg or slice of cheese, dry toast (2-4) with fruit jelly or honey Drink plenty of fluids: at least 2 liters during the day
2. The day of the examination	Before 8:00 AM: take four Peristaltine tablets and one 8-g packet of magnesium sulfate dissolved in a glass of sugar water Breakfast (8:00 AM): same as previous day's breakfast Lunch: two slices of dry toast (no butter) with fruit jelly or honey, one hard-boiled egg if desired Drink plenty of fluids: at least 1 liter during the morning Take two atropine capsules ½ h before the examination

Table 1.3. Results of the standard oral preparation in 100 outpatients (preparations not adapted for the clinical symptoms of the patients) [10]

Effects on fecal movement		Quality of the preparation	
Number of bowel movements:			
Less than three	18%	Excellent	64%
Three to five	26%	Good	25%
More than five	56%	Poor	11%

Table 1.4. Cleansing enema technique

Materials	Enema container (2-liter capacity) Stand for container Long tube ($\simeq$ 1.5 m) Clamping forceps 2.5 liters warm water Nozzle
Technique	1. Insertion of the nozzle Patient in lateral decubitus position with thighs flexed. (In this position, the anus is better exposed and it is easier to straighten the angle between the anal canal and the rectum.) Careful insertion of lubricated enema tip after smoothing anal folds. Do not force. Advance the enema tip just a few centimeters in an upward direction. Place the container about 50 cm above the bed. (The tubing should be filled before attaching the enema tip.) 2. Performing the enema With the patient in the supine or prone position, unclamp the tubing and introduce approximately 500 ml. Turn the patient on to the left side (left lateral decubitus). Introduce 500 ml. The patient turns onto the stomach (prone then right lateral decubitus). Introduce 500 ml. Return the patient to the supine position and introduce the remaining enema.

N. B. Speed is not a factor of effectiveness. However, turning of the patient, as well as the quantity of water needed to fill the colon correctly, are essential. (Turning the patient helps the enema reach the hepatic flexure.)

In the case of colic with sensations of imminent evacuation, do not clamp the tubing. Lower the container in order to allow drainage and prevent flooding. When the colic has passed, continue the enema. The enema should be retained for at least 10 min. If the patient is severely constipated, repeat the enema.

1.1.2.2 Hospitalized Patients

A cleansing enema is necessary to complete the preparation and low-residue diet (Table 1.4). The enema is administered by qualified personnel in the Radiology Department. It is given under low pressure (e.g., set 30–60 cm above the patient's bed) with 2.5 liters of warm water (see Table 1.4). The patient is asked to hold the enema for 10 min and then evacuate as completely as possible. The appearance of the released liquid is noted. If stools are present a second enema is necessary. The examination can be carried out ½ h later. We prescribe atropine sulfate orally ½ h before the examination.

In the case of persistent constipation, the length of the diet and laxative dosage, as well as the number of preparatory enemas, should be increased. If evolutive colitis (Crohn's disease, ulcerative colitis) is suspected, laxative dosage may be reduced or omitted. The low-residue diet and possibly the cleansing enema, carefully administered the night before, should, however, be maintained.

For incontinent, patients the best solution is to use an oral preparation. We do not have sufficient experience in whole-gut irrigation techniques.

1.2 Barium Preparation

In order to be adherent, the barium must be dense and somewhat viscous. We now recommend the use of undiluted barium sulfate (Micropaque from Nicholas Laboratories, 74240 Caillard, France), warmed before use. Most of the radiographs in this study were obtained with Micropaque added to a solution of gum arabic [10]. This results in a lower risk of flocculation, but barium adherence is slightly reduced. It is very suitable for the training of new radiologists. The addition of trimebutine (Debridat, Jouveinal Laboratories, 94260 Fresnes, France) (three vials) to the barium lowers the risk of flocculation [6]. An antifoam silicone (Rhodorsil Prolabo Laboratories, 75015 Paris, 12 Rue Pelée, France) is essential for inhibiting giant bubble formation.

1.3 Material

The material is similar to that used for a standard barium enema. It includes a barium container and its tubing, which is attached to a plastic nozzle. After the colon is partially filled, the nozzle is clamped and separated from the tubing. (At this point, drainage is possible if necessary.) The nozzle is then joined to a 50-cm rubber or plastic tube to which is attached a large insufflation bulb. Insufflation can then begin. Use of a pressurized injector device, (1) which can be completely sterilized, will shorten the examination time (Fig. 1.1).

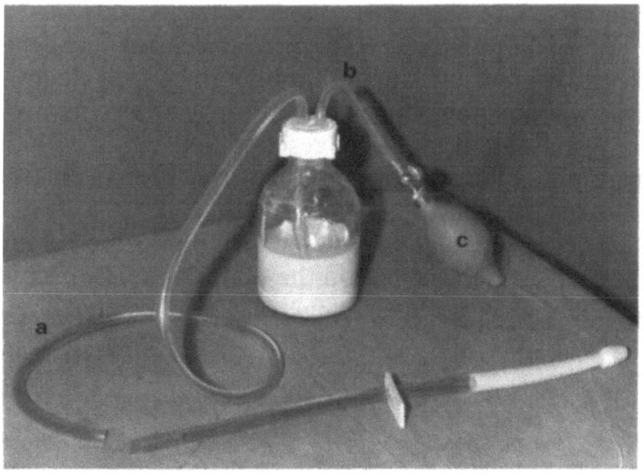

Fig. 1.1. Injection apparatus for double contrast enema. Tube **a** with the rectal nozzle extends to the bottom of the flask. It is this tube that transports the barium. Tube **b** with the insufflation bulb **c** is used for increasing pressure in the flask

1.4 Radiologic Examination

1.4.1 Objectives

The objective of this section is to better acquaint the practitioner and the specialist with the technique and its diagnostic potential:

1. The practitioner should know the contraindications (description of the technique is secondary, but may, however, enable the practitioner to better analyze the radiographs and understand certain contraindications).

2. The specialist should, after memorizing and understanding the described technique, (a) be able to achieve a satisfactory technical level rapidly, after having observed several examinations, (b) especially be able to resolve any problems related to clinical and anatomic abnormalities (dolichocolon, spasms, etc.), and (c) be able to detect possible contraindications. This is an essential part of the specialist's training, another being the interpretation.

1.4.2 Preliminary Procedure

The examination is always preceded by:

1. A short interview, which will verify that the preparation was correctly carried out according to the instructions and ascertain the preparation's effect on fecal movement. (If there have been less than three liquid bowel movements, the oral preparation is insufficient and a cleansing enema should be administered.)

2. A plain abdominal X-ray to check for fecal stasis. If the preparation has clearly been insufficient or thought to be so, a cleansing enema should be given. This will postpone the examination by approximately 2 h. If this is not possible, the examination should be rescheduled, either with the same instructions if they were not followed correctly or with different instructions if the original ones were insufficient.

3. The partial filling phase, which marks the beginning of the examination. If fecal stasis, unobserved on the plain X-ray, is discovered, the enema should be stopped. It is useless, dangerous, and costly to examine a poorly prepared colon.

1.4.3 Procedure

The actual examination has three parts: partial filling, insufflation, and radiographic study.

1.4.3.1 Partial Filling of the Colon (Fig. 1.2)
For opacification of the sigmoid, the patient is first placed in the supine (or prone) position and then turned to the left lateral decubitus position. As soon as the barium reaches the iliac crest, the tube is clamped (see Sect. 1.3). Under fluoroscopy, the opacification of the descending colon and accumulation of bar-

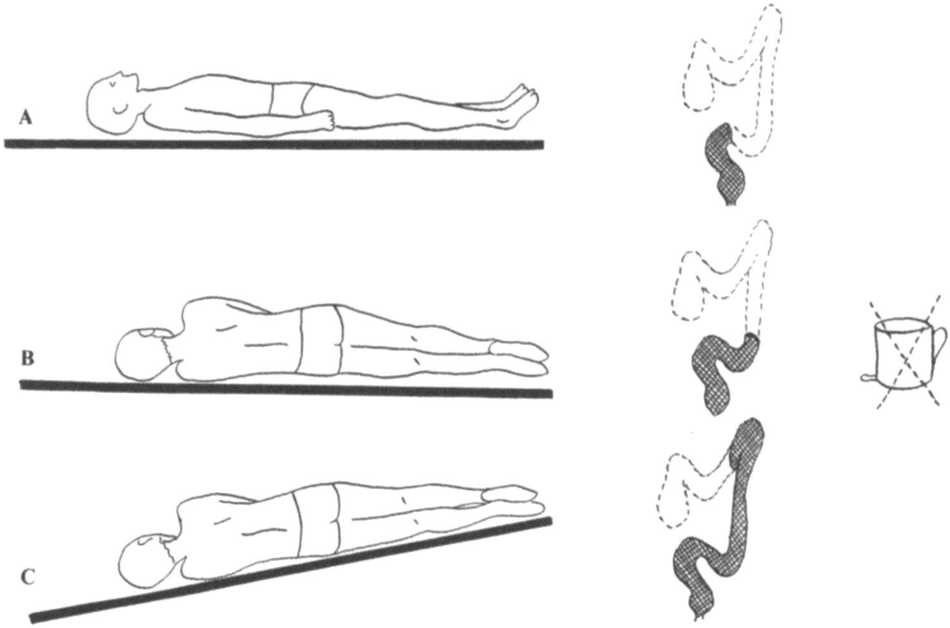

Fig. 1.2. First phase: partial filling. **A,** supine position - filling to top of the sigmoid; **B,** left lateral decubitus - progression to the iliac crest and the tube is clamped; **C,** Trendelenburg's and left lateral decubitus position - barium fills the splenic flexure (if incomplete, filling is resumed). Barium rounds the splenic flexure: the tube is changed

ium in the splenic flexure is followed. (This is facilitated by tilting the table to Trendelenburg's position.) If there is enough barium in the splenic flexure (even if underlying segments are empty) air can now be insufflated. If there is insufficient barium, filling is resumed (some barium will subsequently be drained from the rectum when the splenic flexure is correctly opacified).

Approximately 300 ml barium is used. Less will be needed when the colon is shorter, the progression more rapid, and the radiologist's experience greater. An immediate intravenous injection of glucagon is necessary if spasms occur.

With the splenic flexure filled and the patient in the left lateral decubitus and Trendelenburg's position, air can now be insufflated after attaching a short tube fitted with a bulb.

1.4.3.2 Insufflation (Fig. 1.3)

Insufflation begins using the bulb and under fluoroscopic control. Only very small quantities of air (one or two bulbfuls) are necessary. With the patient in the left lateral decubitus and Trendelenburg's position, air accumulates in the rectosigmoid and pushes the barium column forward. When the column rounds the splenic flexure, the patient turns to the prone position in order to fill the transverse colon and then rapidly turns to the right lateral decubitus position. The table is returned to the horizontal position. Air is again insufflated and barium reaches the hepatic flexure. The insufflated air accumulates in the left

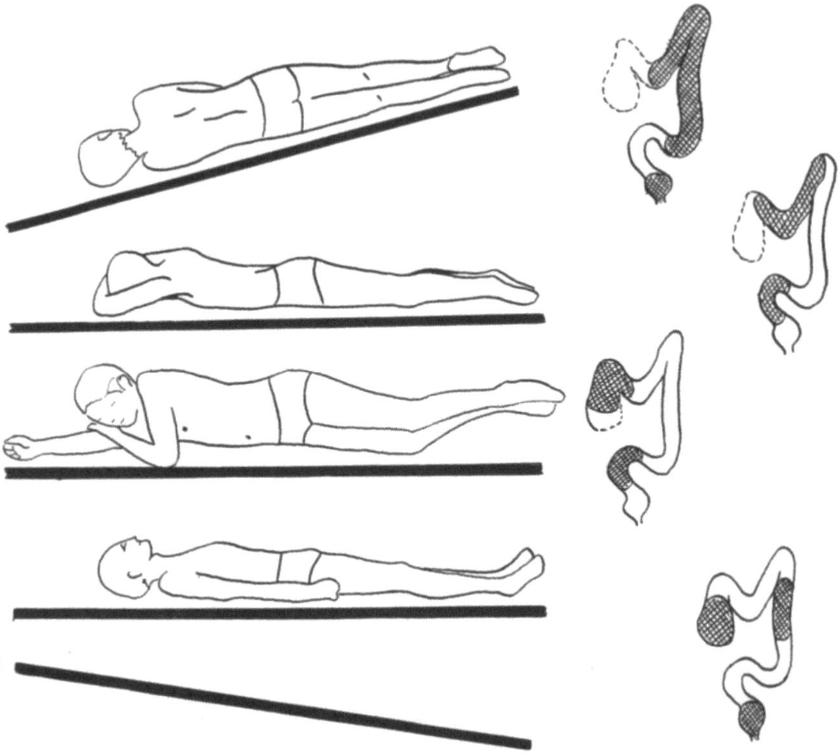

Fig. 1.3. Second phase: Insufflation. **D,** still in the left lateral decubitus and Trendelenburg's position - limited insufflation (only two bulbfuls, to advance the barium column); **E,** patient rapidly turns to the prone position - opacification of the transverse colon; **F,** right lateral decubitus - barium fills the hepatic flexure. Insufflation resumes; **G,** supine position and opacification of the cecum; **H,** table is partially elevated for complete filling of the cecum - insufflation continues and the patient turns completely around. The rectum is drained if necessary

colon. After the patient turns to the supine position and the head of the table is raised 45° if necessary, barium will fill the cecum. The insufflation is continued by having the patient turn around (in the same direction) until good colonic distention is achieved.

1.4.3.3 Radiographic Study

This is carried out under a low kilovoltage (80-90 kV) except for the rectal profile (120-130 kV). The first radiographs are obtained of the sigmoid. If necessary, this is done during insufflation in order to avoid a potentially obscuring ileal reflux. These radiographs include:

1. Table in the horizontal position

a) 24 × 30 cm of the rectosigmoid in the prone right anterior oblique position, if necessary using a balloon and inclined beam
b) 24 × 30 cm of the lateral rectosigmoid
c) 24 × 30 cm of the rectosigmoid in the decubitus, left posterior oblique position with compression

d) 36 × 43 cm in the supine position (with compression for obese patients)
e) 36 × 43 cm in the prone position
f) Views of the cecum can be obtained at this point if it is well coated. A 24 × 30 cm area divided in half is used in the decubitus left and right posterior oblique position and completed, if necessary, by prone views with compression (Trendelenburg's position may, as does the left posterior oblique position, improve cecal distention).

2. Table in vertical position (after being slowly uprighted)
a) 36 × 43 cm, anteroposterior with compression or posteroanterior
b) 30 × 40 cm lengthwise of the splenic flexure and decending colon in right posterior oblique position (or posteroanterior in left anterior oblique position)
c) 30 × 40 cm widthwise of the hepatic flexure and ascending colon in the left posterior oblique position (or posteroanterior in the right anterior oblique position).

3. *In some cases,* in the *vertical position* we can obtain:
a) A 24 × 30 cm radiograph of the sigmoid in the left posterior oblique position plus compression.
b) A 24 × 30 cm lateral radiograph of the rectosigmoid.
c) Radiographs in the lateral decubitus position with a horizontal beam, depending on the equipment. These are useful but not indispensable.

The patient then lies down and all the radiographs are studied. All obscured areas are reexamined with the proper incident angles. Each colonic segment should be clearly visible. Particular attention should be focused on the iliosigmoid junction, where barium often stagnates, as well as the ascending colon. The resulting contrast should be such that the frontal view (opacity of the intermarginal aspect) is visible but much less dense than the mucosal line and haustral folds. *Blurred radiographs should be retaken,* as the definition should be perfect. The patient is free to leave when the radiographs are judged to be satisfactory.

1.4.3.4 Comments

Several points or technical aspects should be emphasized:

1. With atropine, insufflation is *always painless if gently carried out.* Use of a bulb makes it possible to feel any resistance. To use force would cause pain. It suffices to move the patient in order to better distribute the air thus reducing any resistance, before continuing insufflation. *Tolerance of the examination is excellent. The double contrast enema is not a painful examination.*

2. Initial use of too much barium can be remedied by rectosigmoid drainage at the beginning of insufflation. Eventual accumulation of barium in the right colon requires emptying. For this the patient is turned in the opposite direction from that used for filling [from right lateral decubitus to prone (Trendelenburg's position); then from left lateral decubitus to decubitus (horizontal table)]. This movement will empty the right colon, which will appear better insufflated.

3. Flooding of the small bowel can be avoided by placing the patient in the prone position as soon as the barium reaches the cecum. In this position, the ileocecal valve is situated above the barium [7].

4. Exaggerated colonic motility always occurs with diverticulosis, especially at the sigmoid level. Presence of multiple haustral clefts may make interpretation difficult. For this reason it is best to obtain radiographs of the sigmoid when the air is first insufflated. At this point, distention is maximum and the small bowel is not yet opacified.

5. As a general rule, the faster the examination is performed, the better the results. Any prolongation may result in drying of the barium, the radiologic density of which will increase; cracking or flaking of the barium film, making interpretation impossible; and an increase in the number of haustra, making interpretation difficult. These problems vary considerably between patients. The examination is usually not much longer than a well-performed standard examination, taking about 30 min for an experienced radiologist to carry out a problem-free examination.

6. Incontinence is not a contraindication for the technique. When there is sufficient sphincter tonus (easily tested by rectal palpation), continence of the enema and air is generally satisfactory providing the air is gently insufflated. If the sphincter is atonal, water-inflated, large-caliber urinary-type catheters (Foley catheter) may be used. We do not use larger, more rigid balloon catheters due to the risk of possible rectal trauma while moving the patient.

7. For patients with a colostomy, we use a flexible double-balloon catheter especially made for this purpose (Fig. 1.4). This results in satisfactory continence and makes it possible for the patient to turn. Insertion should be nontraumatic and the distal balloon only slightly inflated (several cubic centimeters). It need only block the colostomy orifice, against which it will be pressed by inflation of the proximal balloon (Fig. 1.5). The pathway of the colostomy should have already been determined by digital exploration. A conical irrigation device (Abbott Laboratories, Abbott Pavlz, North Chicago, Illinois 60064, USA) for colostomies can also be used (3).

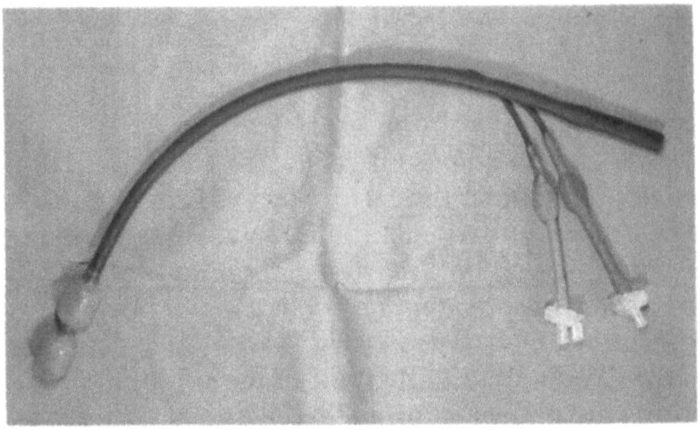

Fig. 1.4. Double balloon catheter for colostomy patients

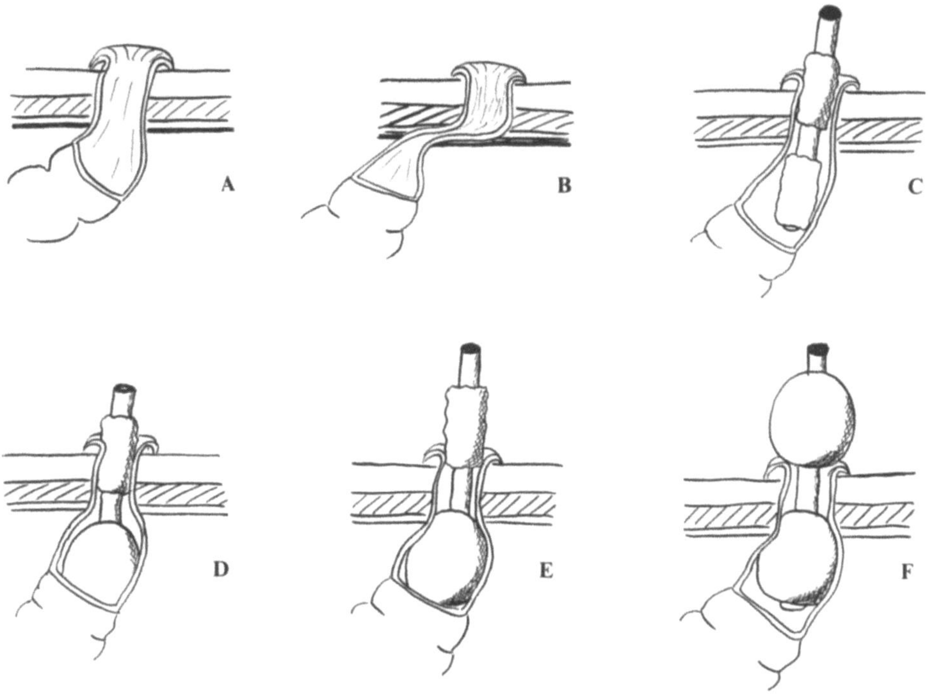

Fig. 1.5. Insertion of the colostomy catheter. **A,** diagram of a colostomy; **B,** finger catherization of the opening is necessary in order to detect a possible "zigzag" pathway which may lead to failure of the catherization or partial trauma; **C,** careful insertion of the catheter, balloon deflated; **D,** slow inflation (several milliliters of water) of the distal balloon; **E,** Inflation stops as soon as the balloon remains in place in the opening despite attempts to remove it by gentle traction of the catheter; **F,** The opening is sealeled by inflation of the external balloon, which then exerts pressure against the internal balloon.
N. B. At the end of the examination, the enema container is lowered to drain the barium and prevent any "leaks" when the catheter is removed. Each step should be gently and painlessly performed. A small flexible urinary catheter is used in the case of stenosis of the opening

1.5 Contraindications

Contraindications are the same for all barium examinations: toxic megacolon and acute diverticulitis. To these we can add evolutive occlusion syndromes, incapacitated patients, and recent rectal biopsies (8-14 days). Contrary to popular belief, insufflation is not dangerous if gently performed. Diverticulosis is not a contraindication.

1.6 Complications

Out of 60000 examinations, Welin [15] reported two cases of perforation of the rectal wall by direct contact of the nozzle and none by overpressure. In both cases there was no passage of barium into the retroperitoneal space. The only problems we encountered in more than 12000 examinations were fainting sensations related to strong air distention when changing to the upright position. This rarely occurs and is without harmful side effects, providing the patient is forewarned of its possible occurrence and asked to report immediately any fainting sensation when in the upright position. The patient must then be supported and the table immediately returned to the horizontal position.

1.7 Conclusion

The technique is simple, but different from the standard technique. It may require a slightly longer training period than for traditional radiology. Lack of adequate training may result in barium flooding, incomplete coating of the colon, bypassing the barium with the air, and severe flocculation. These problems may discourage the new radiologist. They are not due to the technique but to lack of experience. With this in mind and in order to shorten the training period to a minimum, learning the double contrast enema should be carried out intensively on outpatients (whose preparation is easier), and after having observed a number of examinations performed by a radiologist qualified in this technique.

References

1. Ben Mansour A, Sitbon JR, Weissman A, Grellet J (1980) Dispositif injecteur pour mucographie colique. J Radiol 61: 549–550
2. Bret P, Piante M (1972) Radiologie colique en double contraste. Technique de routine. Acta Radiol 15: 637–644
3. Burhenne, HJ (1975) Technique of colostomic examination. Radiology 97: 183–185
4. Hamelin L, Hurtebise M (1971) Le lavement baryté en double contraste. Aspect technique. Union Med Canada 100: 1572–1580
5. Laufer I (1972) Double contrast gastrointestinal radiology with endoscopic correlation. WB Saunders pp 494–506
6. Louvet H, Salas H, Maffioli C, Mesmin F (1979) Intérêt de la trimébutine en radiologie colique en double contraste. Inhibition de la floculation barytée. Acta Endosc 9: 131–146
7. Miller RE (1980) La radiologie du colon. Le lavement baryté. J Radiol 61: 219–225
8. Roussel J, Regent D, Bigard MA (1976) Radiologie digestive en double contraste. Masson, Paris
9. Weissman A, Clot M, Grellet J (1978) Note de technique: réalisation pratique du double contraste colique. J Radiol Electrol 59: 299–302
10. Weissman A, Labayle D, Clot M, Grellet J (1977) Préparation ambulatoire au lavement en double contraste: étude rétrospective sur 100 malades non hospitalisés. J Radiol Electrol 58: 441–444
11. Weissman A, Grellet J (1979) Sonde pour exploration radiologique des colostomisés par lavement en double contraste. J Radiol 60: 315–316
12. Welin S (1958) Modern trends in diagnostic roentgenology of the colon. The Mackenzie Davidson Memorial lecture. Brit Jour Radiol 369: 453–464
13. Welin S (1971) Examination and cleansing of the large bowel. J Belge Radiol 54: 1–6
14. Welin S (1974) New diagnostic technic. The superiority of double contrast radiology. Dis Colon and Rectum 17: 13–20
15. Welin S, Welin G (1976) The double contrast examination of the colon. Experiences with the Welin modifications. Thieme, Stuttgart

2 Interpretation (General Rules, Normal and False Images)

Interpretation of the double contrast barium enema is fundamentally different from that of the single contrast enema. New rules of interpretation, which must be fully understood, are necessary in that more and particularly different kinds of information are provided by double contrast.

2.1 General Rules of Interpretation

Two points are fundamental: (1) Radiologic appearances of the colon depend on the quantity of air and barium used and the formation mechanism of the image. (2) Spatial configuration of the colon and the patient's position play a determining role in the distribution of air and barium.

2.1.1 Different Radiologic Aspects of the Colon and the Formation Mechanism of the Image

Using a vertical beam on a patient in the horizontal position, the colon may have three different appearances (Figs. 2.1, 2.2). It may be insufflated and coated with a fine film of barium. This is the actual double contrast image (Figs. 2.1, 2.2 A). It may be insufflated and contain a small quantity of barium (a movable pool in its lowest or most dependent segment). It may be filled with barium (or appear so) due to a large quantity of barium obscuring the entire intermarginal aspect (Figs. 2.1, 2.2 C, D).

2.1.1.1 Actual Double Contrast Image

The image is derived from the film of barium which uniformly coats the mucosa. This opacity can be increased by three different effects:

Tangent Effect (Fig. 2.3). When the incident beam is tangent to a curved surface covered with barium, a dense and regular line appears. This effect results in the formation of border lines and the image of haustral folds which protrude into the lumen.

Addition Effect (Fig. 2.4). When several barium-coated surfaces are superimposed, their radiologic opacities are added. This mechanism comes into play for the intermarginal aspect (frontal double contrast) and even more so for bends, haustral folds, etc.

Accumulation of Barium (Fig. 2.5). Accumulation of barium may be due to gravity in an ulceration or around a raised lesion (Fig. 2.5 A); capillary attraction at the junction of two acute- or even obtuse-angled surfaces (polyps and fecal matter) (Fig. 2.5 B, C); or the junction of two barium-coated surfaces (false images when anterior and posterior aspects of a segment are compressed (Figs. 2.6, 2.7). In general, the resulting images are low in density and homogeneous for the colonic walls. Density increases near the margins, which are marked by a dense regular line. This line also appears for bends and haustral clefts (Figs. 2.8–2.10).

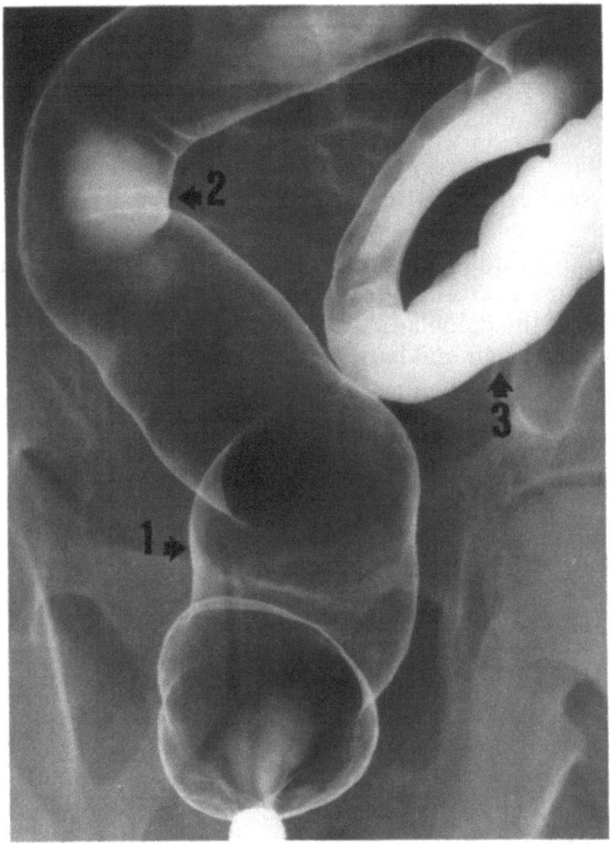

Fig. 2.1. Double contrast appearance of the colonic mucosa. **1,** insufflated segment coated with a fine film of barium. Note the regularity of the border lines and homogeneous character of the colonic mucosa of the walls; **2,** insufflated segment with a barium pool on the dependent surface. Note the blurred margins; **3,** segment apparently filled with barium. The entire intermarginal aspect is obscured

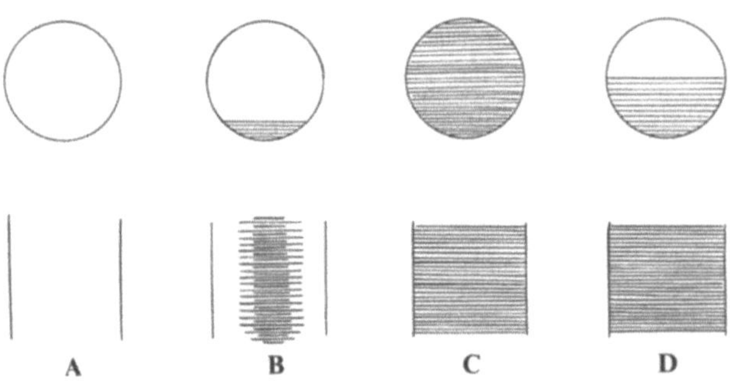

Fig. 2.2 Colonic appearance, depending on the quantity of air and barium in the lumen. **A,** segment insufflated and coated with barium; **B,** a barium pool with blurred edges on the dependent surface; **C,** barium-filled segment; **D,** only partially filled segment but with the same appearance as in C due to high barium density completely obscuring the intermarginal aspect

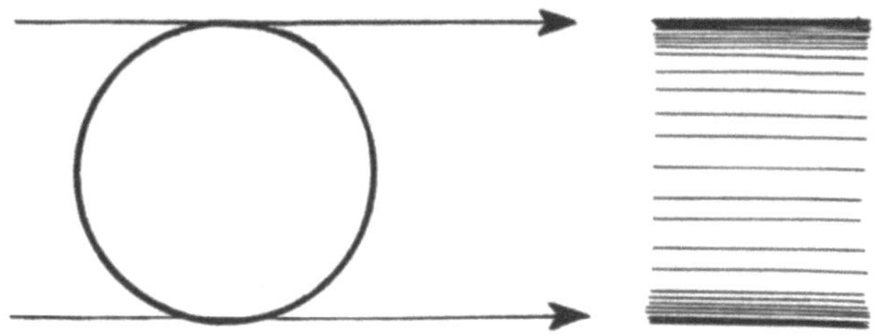

Fig. 2.3. Borderline formation by the tangent effect

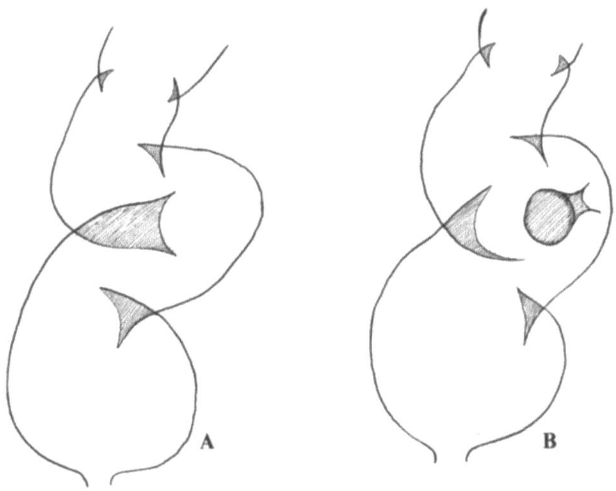

Fig. 2.4. Reinforcement of the radiologic opacity by the addition effect. **A,** density reinforcement occurs for bends and Houston's valves *(darkened areas)*; **B,** the density of barium coating a polyp is added to that of the colonic walls

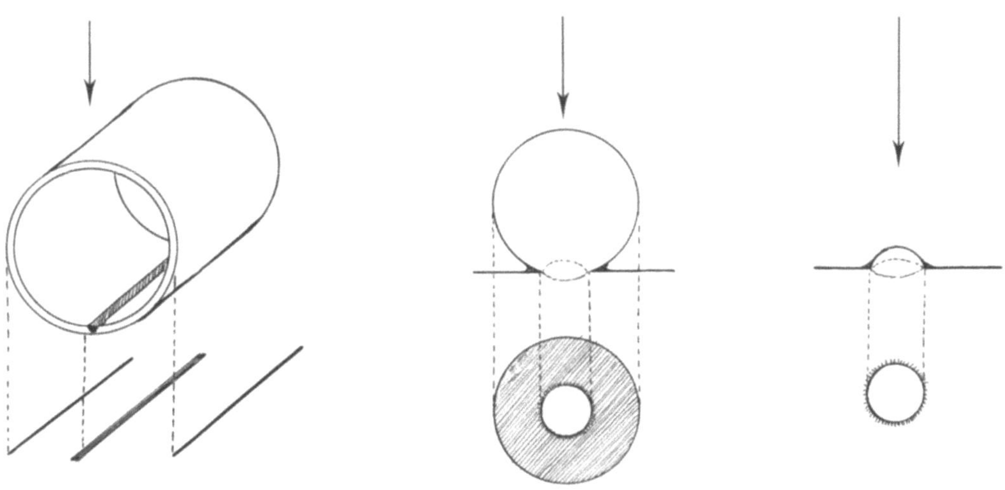

Fig. 2.5. Reinforcement of the radiologic opacity by barium accumulation. **A,** accumulation in an ulceration (longitudinal); **B,** accumulation at the junction of two surfaces (acute angle); **C,** accumulation at the junction of two surfaces (obtuse angle)

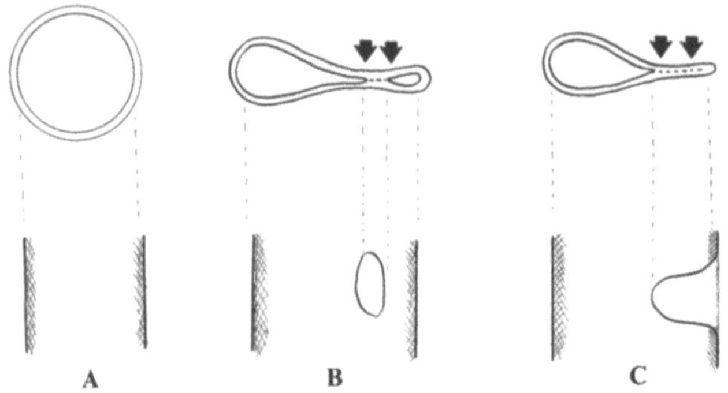

Fig. 2.6. Accumulation at the junction of two barium-coated surfaces; **A,** normal colon; **B,** strong compression brings two walls of a colonic segment into contact; dense line bordering the area of contact appears; **C,** the colonic margin may also be compressed, erasing the margin in question and creating an opaque line which will disappear when compression stops

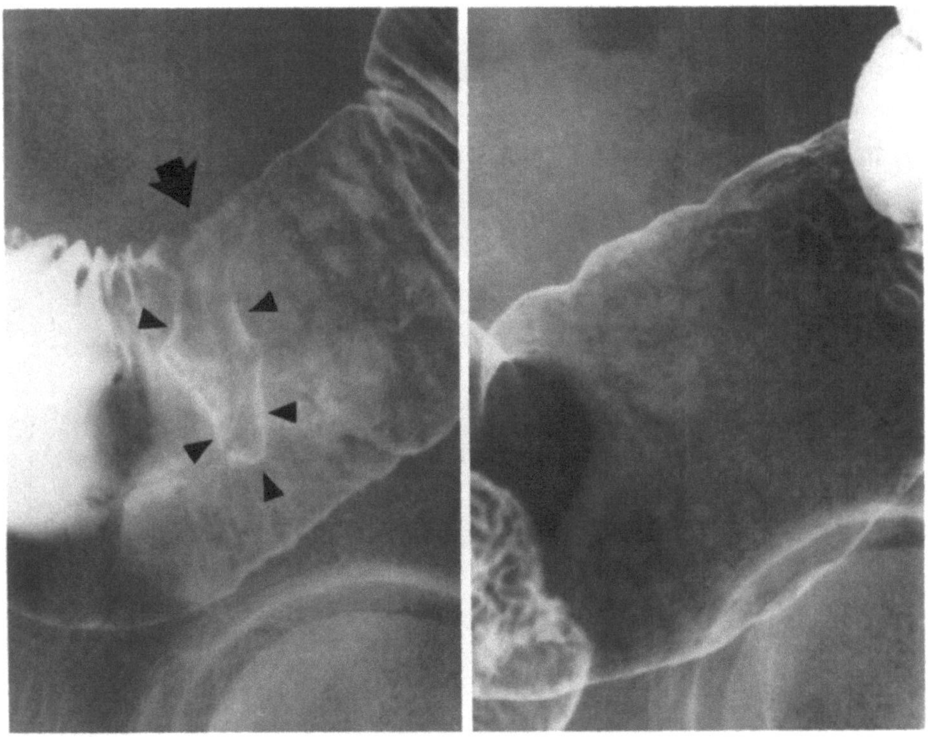

Fig. 2.7. A, example of the image formed by strong compression of the sigmoid *(arrows)*; **B,** the image in **A** disappears when compression stops

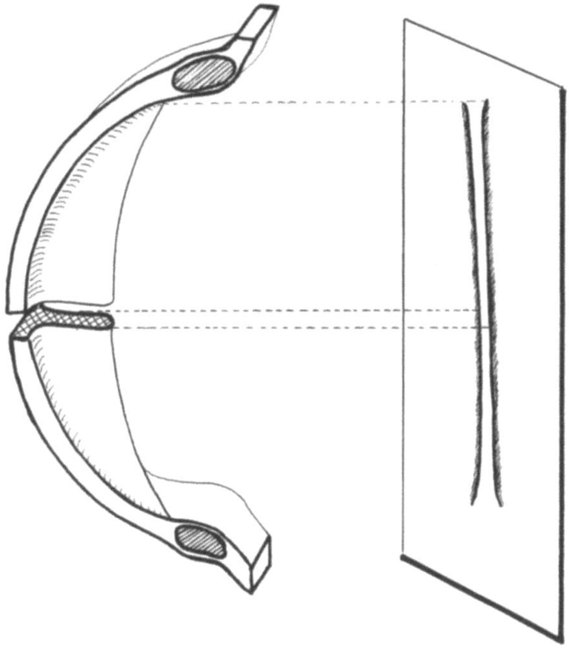

2.8 A

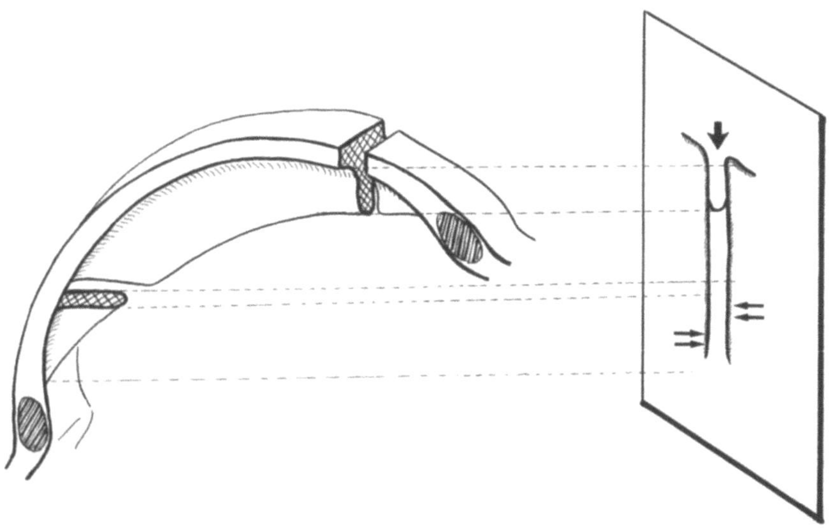

2.8 B

Fig. 2.8. Formation of a colonic valve image. Colonic valves are semilunar folds which lie between the longitudinal bands (see Fig. 8.1) and project into the lumen. **A** When the incident beam is perpendicular to the axis of the colonic segment containing a valve, the resulting frontal image is one of inverted parenthesis (since the incident beam is tangent to both sides of the valve). **B,** The image changes if the valve is not exactly frontal and if its free margin becomes tangent to the incident beam. A medially convex notch forms at the colonic margin *(arrow)* and is extended toward the lumen by two straight lines (*double arrow,* image of the two sides of the valve). Fig. 2.8. C, D see page 18

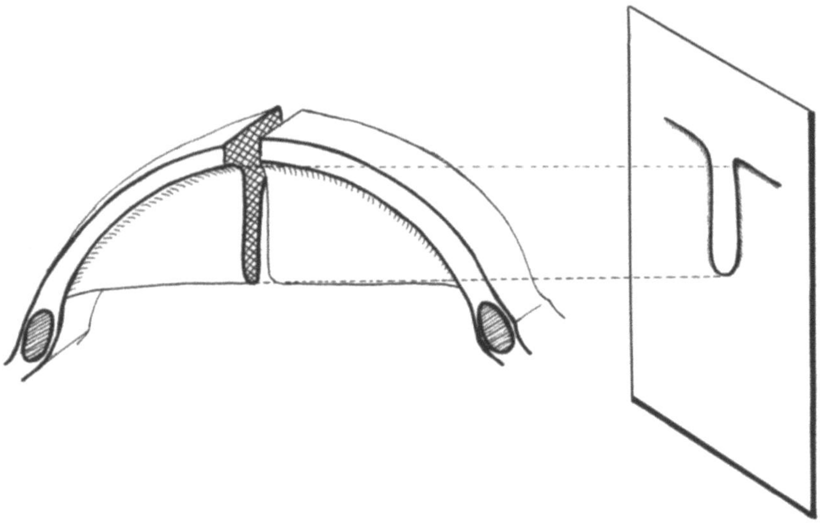

2.8C

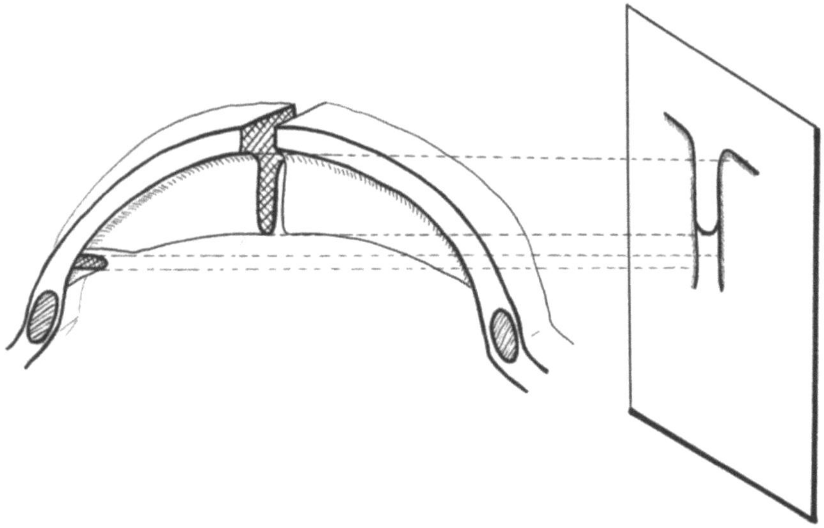

2.8D

Fig. 2.8. Formation of a colonic valve image. **C** When the valve is seen in profile, the resulting image is either that of a "hairpin" notch or **D** a notch extended by two short straight lines which correspond to the extremities of the valves

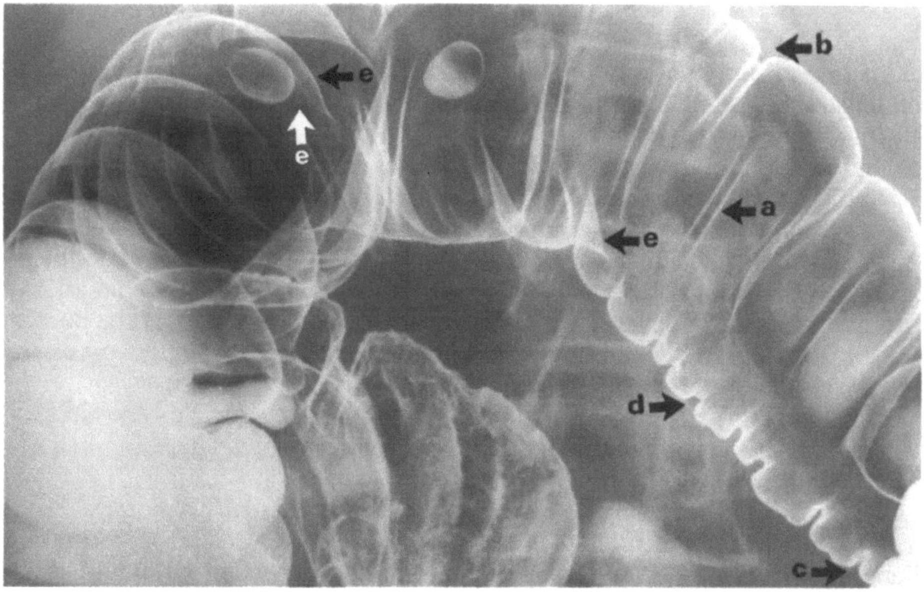

Fig. 2.9. Colonic valves: double contrast image of a colonic segment (right angle). The three rows of colonic valves are clearly seen with different incident beams. **a**, frontal; **b**, three-quarter view; **c**, **d**, profile; **e**, the incident beam is no longer perpendicular to the segment's axis, giving the valves a semilunar appearance. In this case, it is the addition effect that outlines the valve since the incident beam passes throught both surfaces of the colon and valve (four layers of barium)

Fig. 2.10. Colonic valve appearance. The valves appear equally spaced in rows. Some *(arrows)* appear as filling defects (outlined by barium). This makes it possible to identify valves on the dependent surface

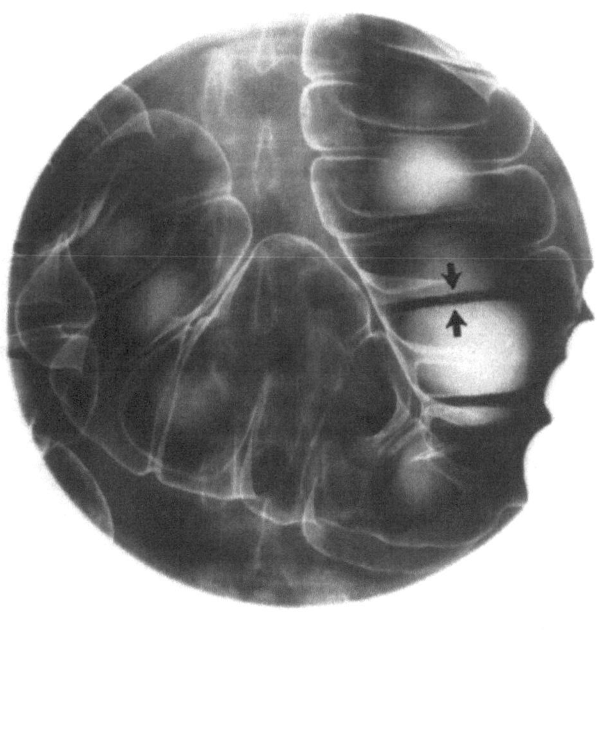

2.1.1.2 Insufflated Segments Containing a Small Amount of Barium (Figs. 2.11, 2.12)

An opaque barium pool can form in the insufflated segments. It is movable, depending on the patient's position, and is found on the most dependent segment. This pool (due to the progressive thinning of barium at the periphery) always has blurred borders except when transversely crossed by a haustral fold (Fig. 2.10). Any interruption or sharp limitation of one of its margins indicates (as does a filling defect) a lesion implanted on the dependent surface of the colonic segment in question (Figs. 2.11 B, 2.13). In addition to its importance in situating the lesion (on the dependent surface), this sign ("pool" sign) has an important diagnostic value in that it may appear for very flat lesions if the pool is thin (Fig. 2.14 C). On the other hand, it is important to note that a pool may partially mask a lesion on the nondependent surface (Figs. 2.14, 2.15).

In summary, the presence of a barium pool may, depending on the circumstances, indicate a lesion or may partially or even completely mask it.

2.1.1.3 If the Colonic Segment Appears Completely Filled With Barium

In this case, traditional rules of interpretation must be used first. If contour changes can be normally analyzed, the intermarginal aspect image should be interpreted, taking two points into account: (1) the filling might be incomplete (Fig. 2.11 D) and (2) the high density of the barium used may mask a lesion or minimize its size. These two possibilities explain why the filling defect for tumoral lesions is not always present and sometimes less evident than with the classic technique.

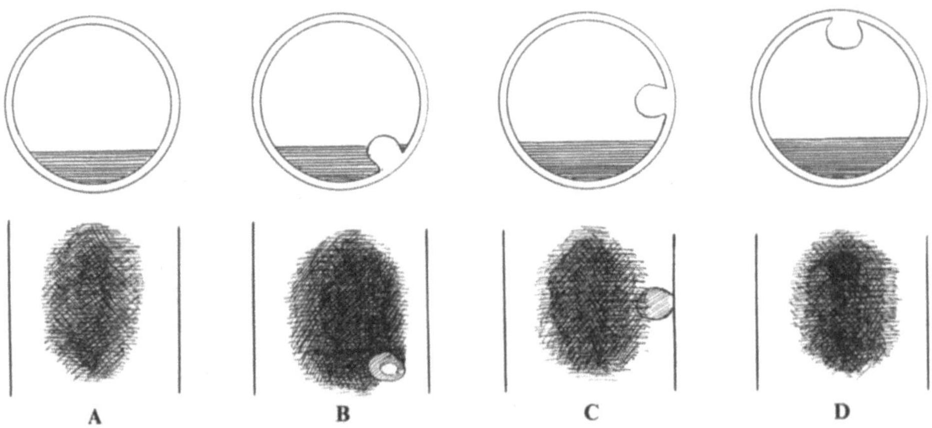

Fig. 2.11. Puddle sign. **A,** normal pool with blurred margins; **B,** a tumor on the dependent surface is seen as a filling defect; **C, D,** a tumor on the nondependent surface is partially (**C**) and totally (**D**) masked by the pool

Fig. 2.12. Montage of Figure 2.11. **A, B, C,** and **D** same as in Fig. 2.11

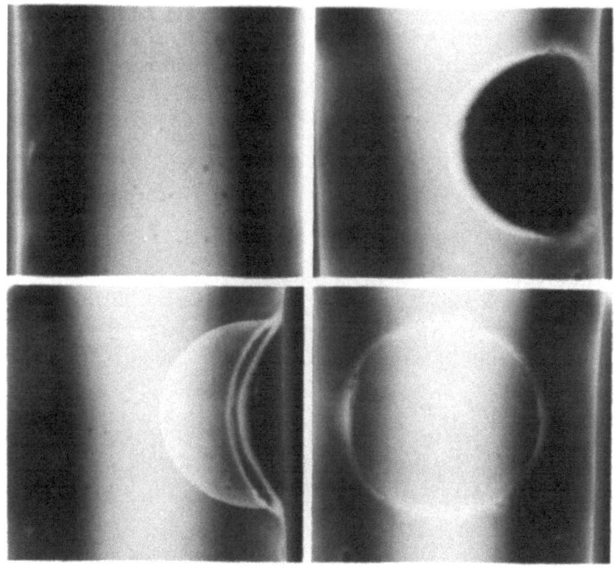

A B C D

Fig. 2.13. Filling defect caused by a tumor on the dependent surface (adenocarcinoma of the sigmoid)

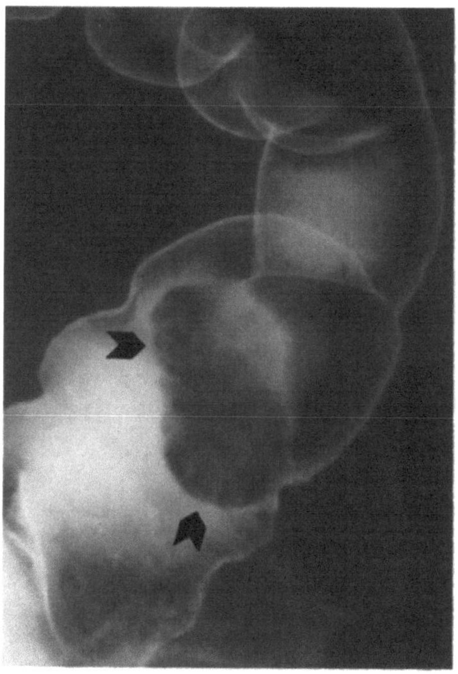

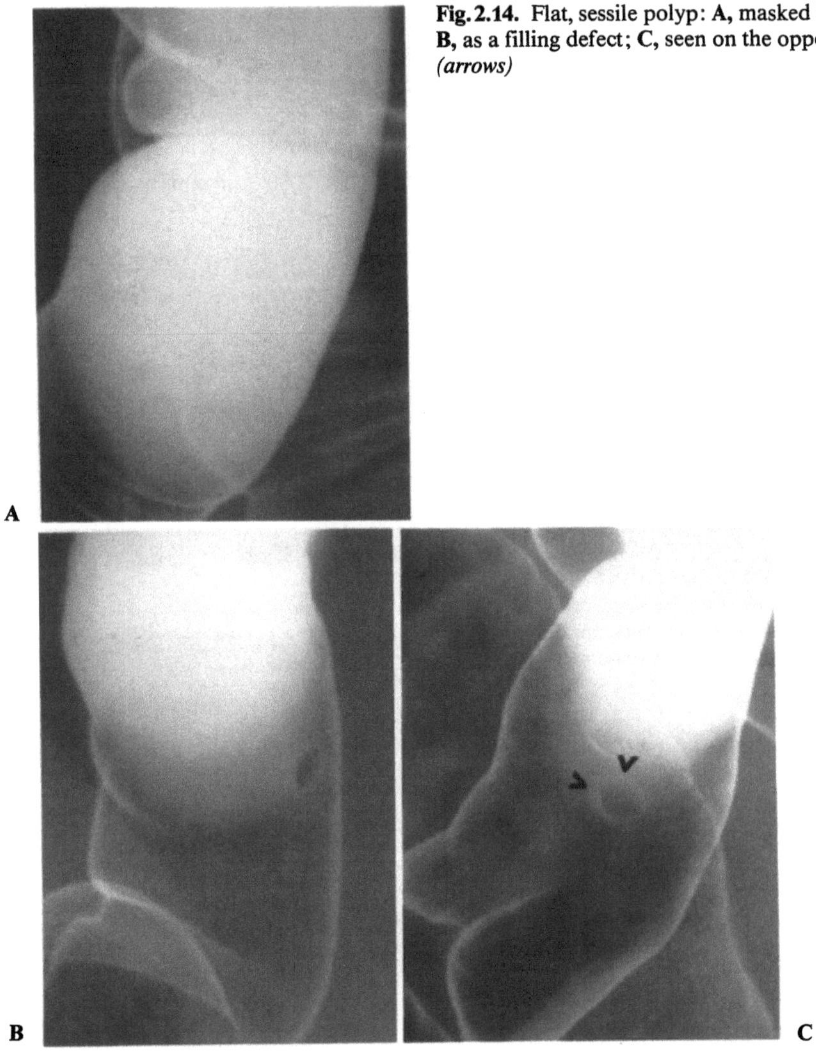

Fig. 2.14. Flat, sessile polyp: **A,** masked by the pool; **B,** as a filling defect; **C,** seen on the opposite wall *(arrows)*

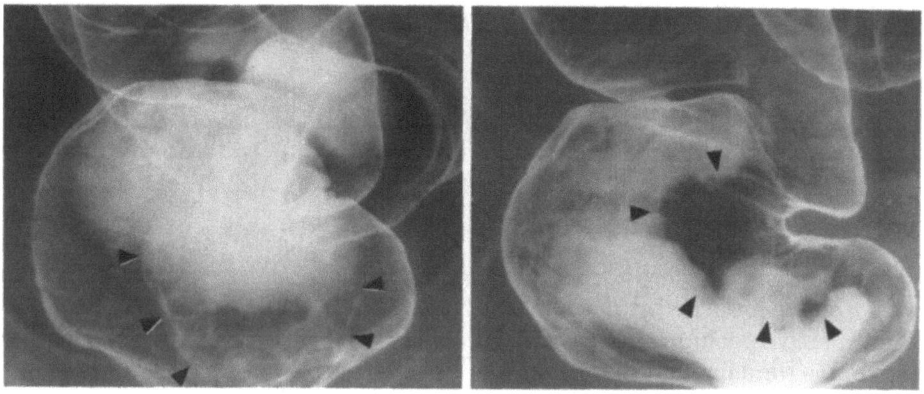

A B

Fig. 2.15. A In the supine position, the tumoral contours are partially masked by the pool. The importance of the filling defect should not be ruled out, but rather viewed according to the patient's change in position. **B** The tumor appears surrounded by barium; the pool is "severed" (radiograph obtained with the patient in the prone position)

Fig. 2.16. Profile diagrammatic representation of the left colon. *white,* free segments; *dotted,* attached segments; **1,** rectum; **2,** sigmoid; **3,** attached descending colon; **4,** descending part of splenic flexure (free); **5,** ascending part of splenic flexure (free)

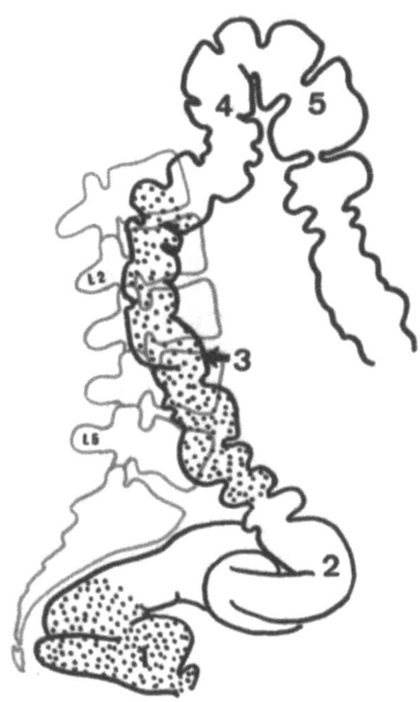

2.1.2 Importance of the Spatial Configuration of the Colon and the Patient's Position for Air and Barium Distribution

If knowledge of colonic anatomy in standard radiology is only needed to better position the flexures and avoid overlapping, it is essential with double contrast in order to carry out and interpret the examination correctly with the new imaging.

2.1.2.1 Anatomic Review: Respective Position of the Different Colonic Segments in the Abdominopelvic Cavity

The respective position of the different colonic segments in an anteroposterior direction is fundamental since, for a patient in a horizontal position, it controls the distribution of barium and air in the colon. The most frequent conformation, but not the only one (5), is easily understood with the aid of frontal and profile diagrams (Figs. 2.17, 2.18).

The cecum is unattached and lies anterior to the ascending colon. The latter passes in a cranial and dorsal direction toward the hepatic flexure. It is maintained in contact with the posterior abdominal wall by the peritoneum.

The transverse colon describes a curve with its convexity pointing in a caudal and ventral direction. Its central segment comes into contact with the anterior abdominal wall. It is attached at the hepatic flexure to the medial border of the descending duodenum (a few centimeters right of the medial line). The remaining two-thirds is movable.

The splenic flexure, which is part of the transverse colon, is also movable. It is often situated quite high in front of the spleen near the left cupola. The ascending segment of the flexure follows the transverse colon without transition and is thus still anterior. Its descending segment is in a caudal and dorsal direction. At the caudal end of the spleen it becomes the descending colon, which is attached posteriorly and laterorachially (Fig. 2.16).

The iliac colon, which follows the descending colon, begins at the iliac crest and is situated against the iliac fossa at a variable level depending on its length. It curves medially and dorsally and ends at the medial border of the iliopsoas. The top of this curve is *anterior to its extremities.*

The sigmoid colon is continuous with the iliac colon and begins at the medial border to the iliopsoas. Its length varies and it describes a long curve before ending anterior to the third sacral vertebra.

The rectum lies in the sacrococcygeal curve. It is caudally and posteriorly concave at its lower extremity.

2.1.2.2 Practical Implications for Analysis of the Radiographs

Following insufflation, the air quickly diffuses throughout the colon and distends the nondependent segments whereas the barium moves to dependent zones. Distribution of barium depends on the colon's spatial configuration in a particular position but varies if the position of the patient changes. This characteristic, which is specific to double contrast, can be used to choose the position best suited for insufflation or opacification of a particular colonic region during the examination. It also enables the specialist, by studying the radiographs, to

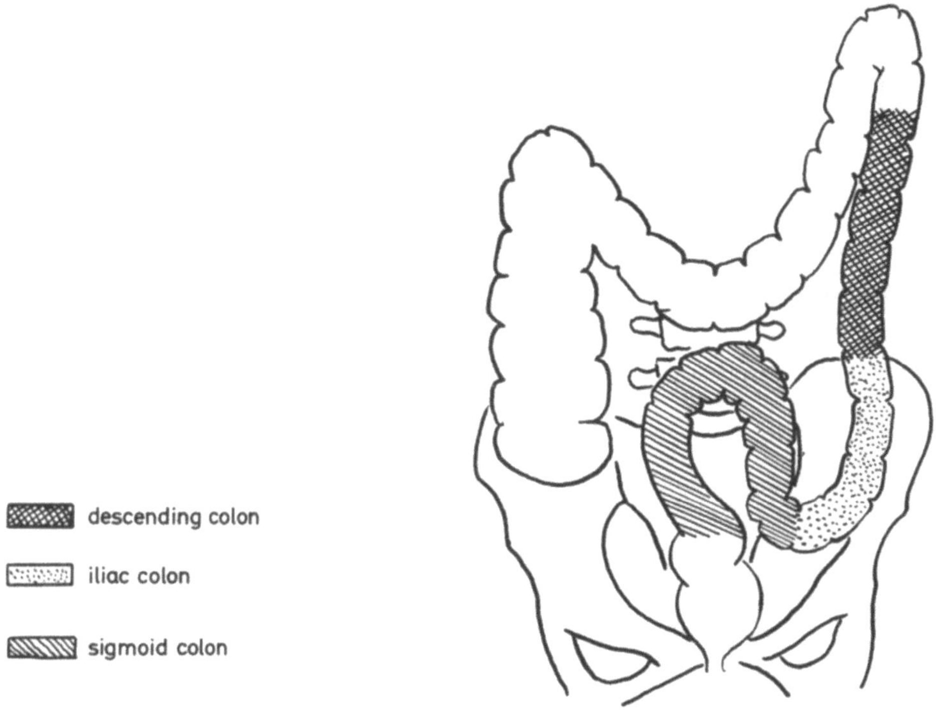

Fig. 2.17. Frontal diagrammatic representation of the colon: a knowledge of the limits between descending, iliac, and sigmoid colons is particularly important

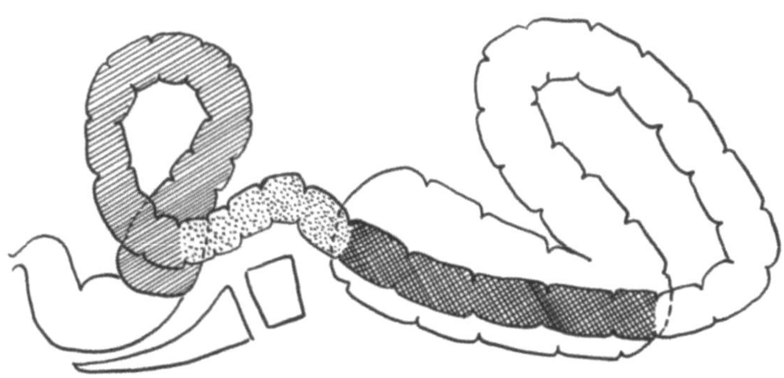

Fig. 2.18. Profile diagrammatic representation of the colon, showing the different segments of the left colon. Note the curve formed by the iliac colon

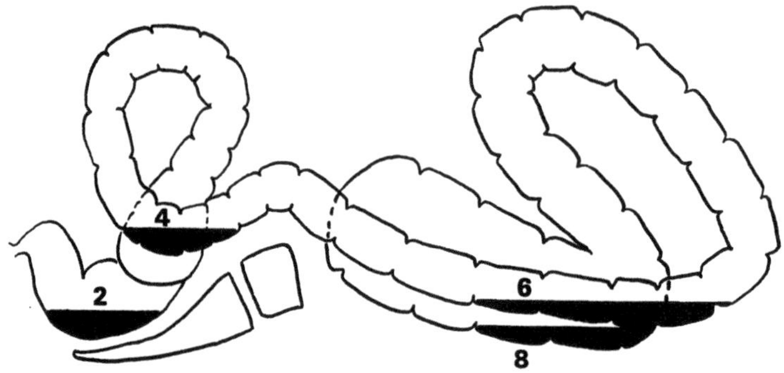

Fig. 2.19. Profile diagrammatic representation of the colon with the patient in the *supine position*. Barium is found in the center of the rectum **(2)** iliosigmoid junction **(4)**, and descending **(6)** and ascending colon **(8)**

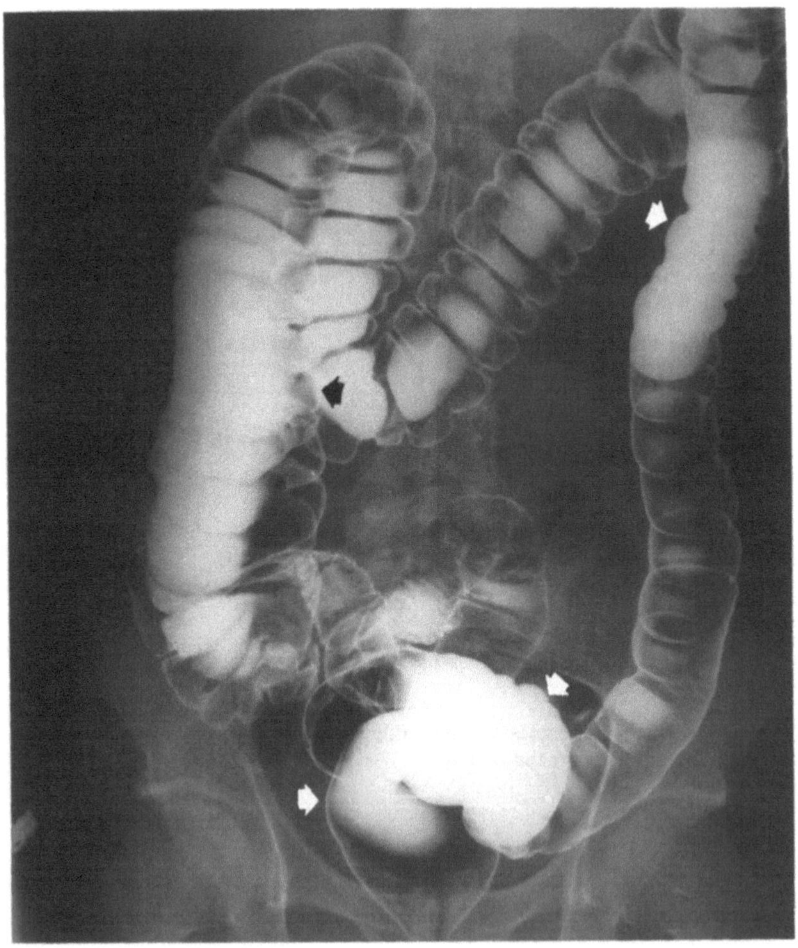

Fig. 2.20. Radiograph taken with the patient in the *supine position*. Barium is again found in the rectum (central part), iliosigmoid junction, and descending and ascending colons *(arrows)*

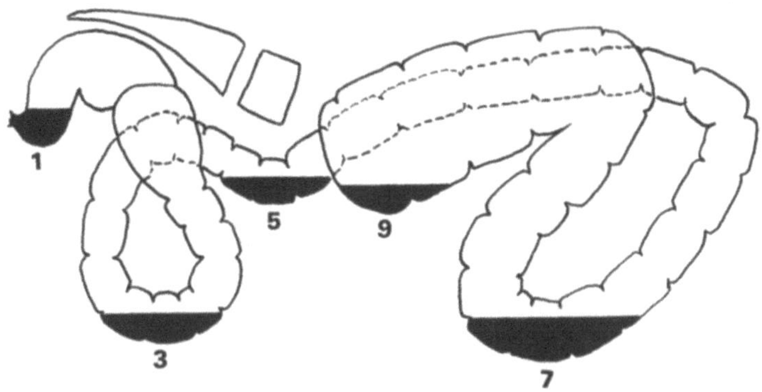

Fig. 2.21. Diagrammatic representation of barium distribution in the colon *(prone position)*. Barium is found in the distal part of the rectum **(1)**, iliac colon **(5)**, transverse colon **(7)**, bas-fond of the cecum (anterior aspect) **(9)**, and, in some cases, top of the sigmoid **(3)**

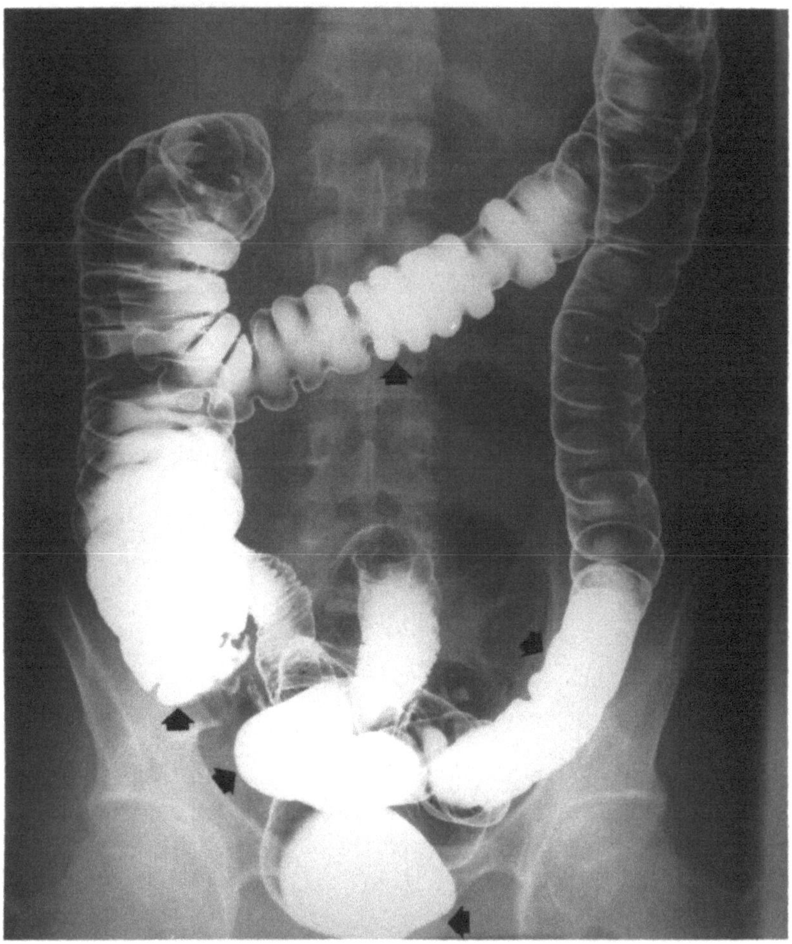

Fig. 2.22. Radiograph obtained with the patient in the *prone position*. Typical barium distribution: distal end of the rectum, top of the sigmoid, iliac, and transverse colons, and bas-fond of the cecum *(arrows)*

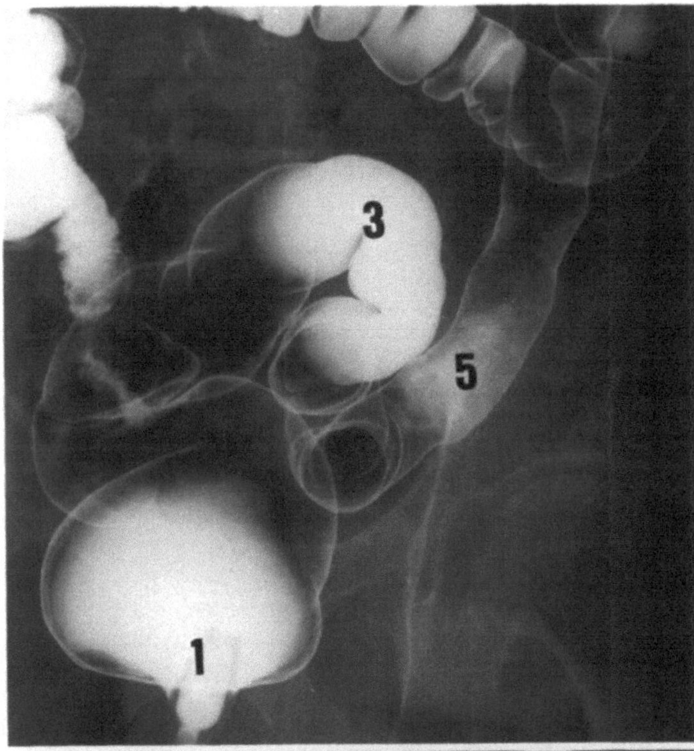

2.23 A

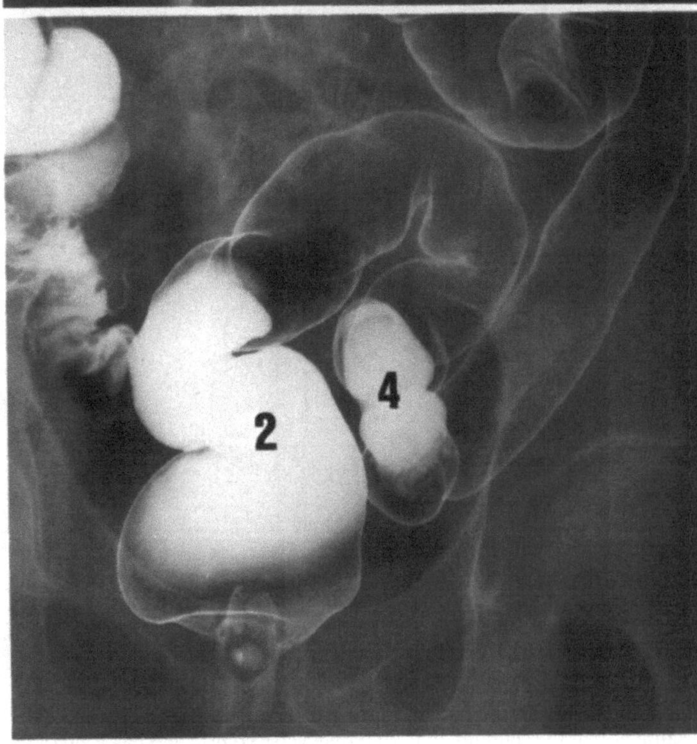

2.23 B

determine from the distribution of the barium the position in which the radiograph was obtained and consequently the exact location of pathological images, or to explain their disappearance (see pool sign).

1. In the supine position with a vertical beam (Figs. 2.19, 2.20, 2.23), pools of barium are found in the most posterior segments: the central section of the rectum, the iliac-sigmoid junction, and the ascending and decending colons near the flexures. The distal end of the rectum, sigmoid loop, iliac colon, transverse colon, and bas-fond of the cecum are well insufflated.

2. In the prone position (Figs. 2.21-2.23), barium is found in the most anterior segments: distal end of the rectum, tops of the sigmoid and iliac colons, transverse colon, and proximal end of the cecum. Those areas opacified in the supine position are now insufflated.

3. In the upright position barium moves to dependent segments of the colon: cecum, central section of the transverse colon, distal section of the descending colon, iliac colon and distal section of the rectum. In this position, the flexures, transverse colon and top of the sigmoid are easily analyzed since they are well distended and cleared of barium and possibly of nonadherent fecal matter. These radiographs are easily recognized from the horizontal fluid levels in dependent zones and haustral cul-de-sacs. (The same is true for radiographs obtained in the lateral decubitus position with a horizontal beam.)

◁ **Fig. 2.23.** Barium distribution in the rectosigmoid according to the patient's position. **A** Radiograph obtained with the patient in the prone right anterior oblique position shows barium in the distal end of the rectum **(1)**, top of the sigmoid loop **(3)**, and iliac colon **(5)**. **B** Radiograph obtained with the patient in the opposite position: supine and slightly left posterior oblique. Air is found in the previously opacified segments and barium in the central part of the rectum **(2)** and iliosigmoid junction **(4)**

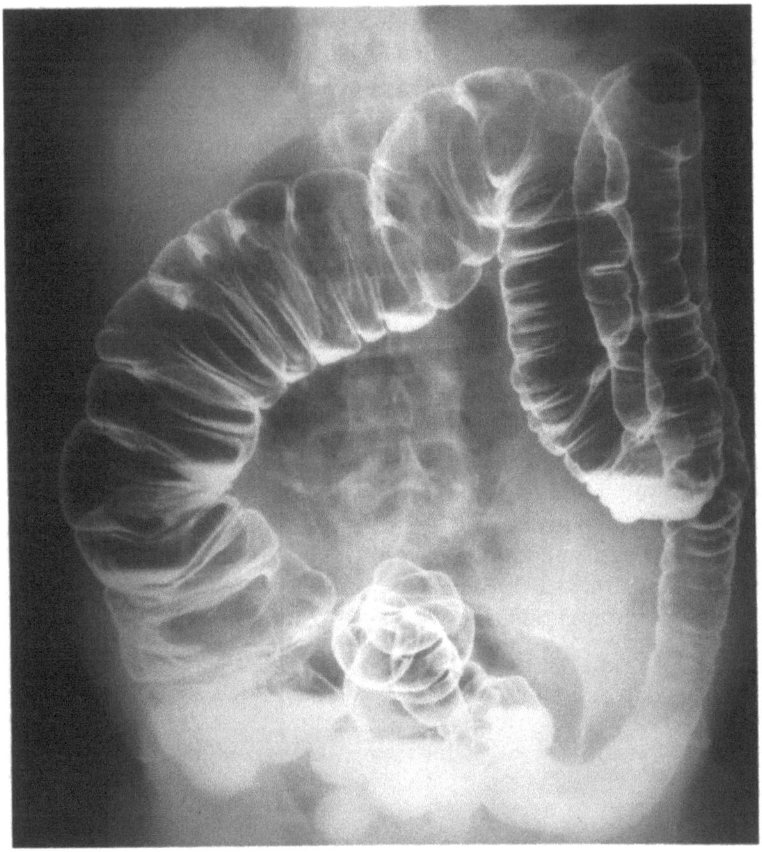

Fig. 2.24. Normal colon: segmental nonpropulsive contractions. Haustral clefts are clearly seen in the right and transverse colons. They are less evident in the descending and sigmoid colons

2.2 Colonic Morphology and Motor Activity

2.2.1 Morphology

Depending on the caliber of the intestine and the number and depth of the haustra, colonic structure does not appear significantly different after insufflation than after a classic single contrast examination. In normal conditions, two appearances may be observed. According to Wolf [11], they signal different physiologic activities.

1. The first appearance is that in which the caliber is normal and the haustral clefts well delineated (segmental nonpropulsive contractions). They are more numerous and deeper in the right and transverse colon than in the descending colon and are much less frequent in the sigmoid (Fig. 2.24). As distention increases, haustral clefts become more shallow. They may vary in number and site

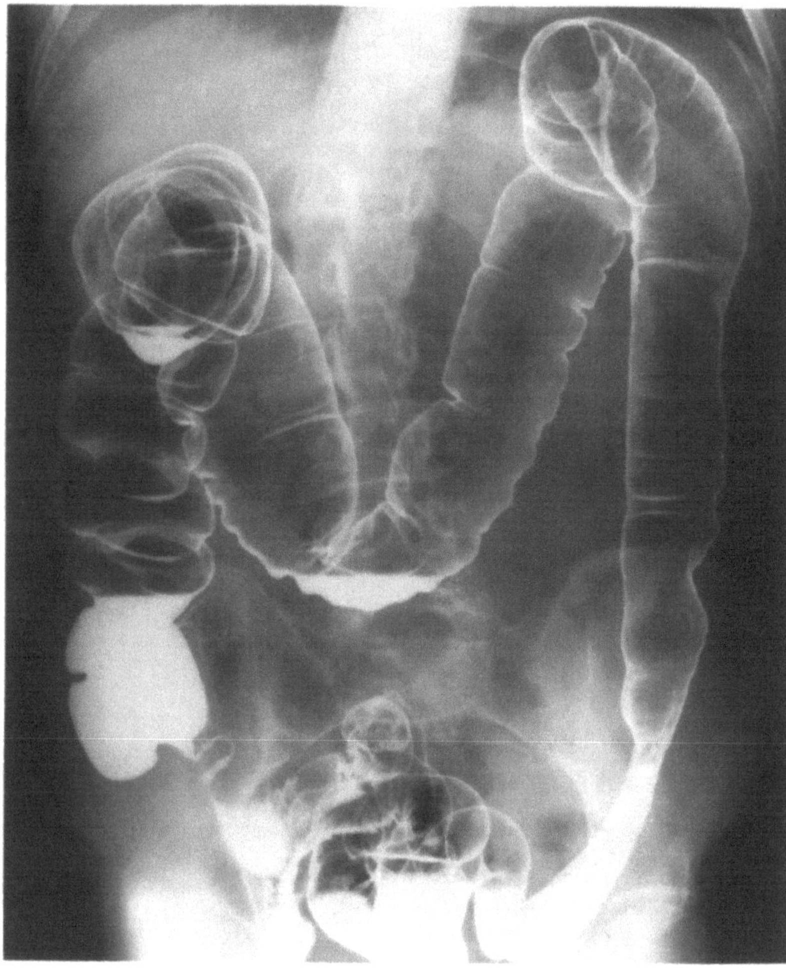

Fig. 2.25. Normal colon: propulsive transport contraction. The caliber remains normal; haustral clefts are much fewer, especially in the left colon

during the examination and tend to become more pronounced if it is prolonged.

2. *The second appearance* (Fig. 2.25), which is seen much less frequently, is where the colon is tubulated with a caliber which is normal but smaller than in the previous case. Haustra are practically nonexistent in the left colon and rare in the right colon. According to Wolf [11], this corresponds to a "propulsive transport contraction." It is important to note that both appearances may be found in the same patient during the same or repeated examinations.

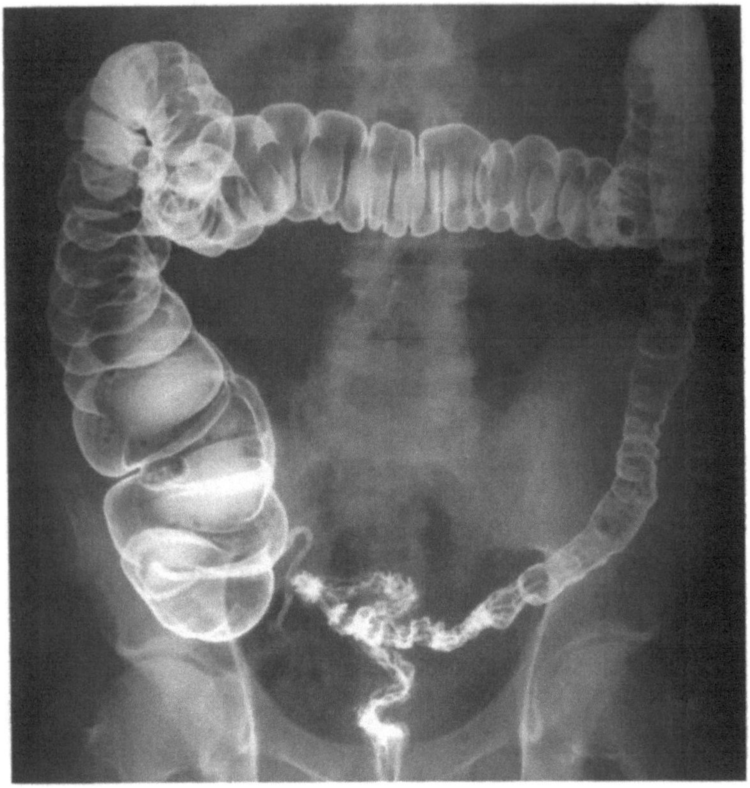

Fig. 2.26. Radiograph obtained after evacuation: here only the rectosigmoid was drained

2.2.2 *Motor Activity*

Insufflation and the use of antispasmodic substances obviously modify the normal motor activity of the colon. Nevertheless, it should be noted that retrograde filling, whether by fluid or air, is antiphysiologic. Thus, nothing prevents us from redefining colonic motor activity as studied by double contrast.

A number of facts have been established: (1) *Obtaining radiographs after evacuation* is generally difficult since drainage is often limited to the sigmoid (Fig. 2.26). (2) *Air displacement* from one segment to another occurs rapidly. Passive collapse of lower segments may occur if insufflation is incomplete: the cecum and descending colon may collapse in the upright position (Figs. 2.27, 2.28) and the transverse colon in the prone position. Overdistention of certain segments is also possible (the cecum at the end of the examination and the flexures in the upright position). Both these problems make interpretation impossible. (3) *Spasms* are rare in normal subjects.

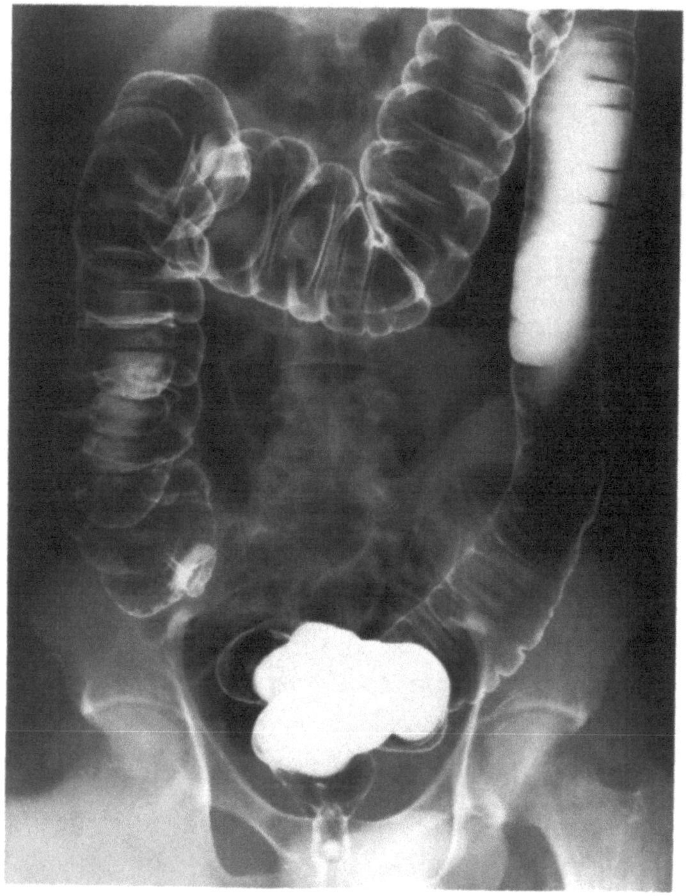

Fig. 2.27. Radiograph of a normal colon taken with the patient in the supine position

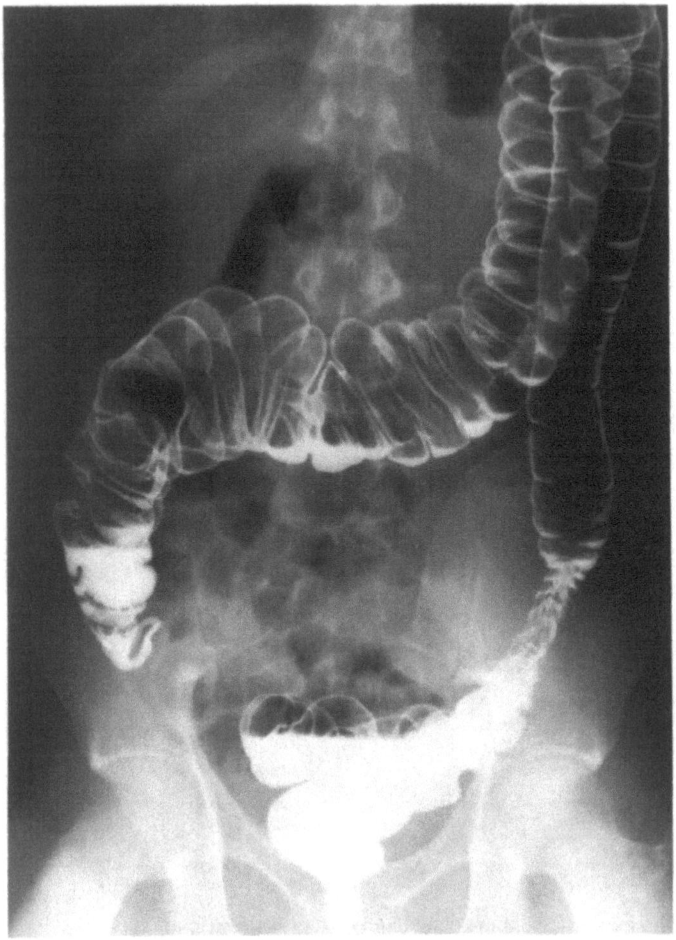

Fig. 2.28. After moving the patient to the upright position, collapse of the dependent segments can be seen - especially the cecum and descending colon (same patient as in Fig. 2.27)

2.3 Normal Appearance of the Colonic Mucosa (Walls and Margins), Physiologic Variants, False Images

Precise evaluation of mucosal relief is one of the advantages of the double contrast enema. This makes possible the early diagnosis of organic colitis and conditions normally undetected by standard radiology (lymphoid nodular hyperplasia, for example). The state of mucosal relief is reflected by the appearance of the barium which coats the colon and appears in the intermarginal aspect (double contrast of the walls) and on the margins and colonic valves (double contrast of the margins). Normally, the appearance of the walls in double contrast is homogeneous. Density increases evenly toward the margins, whose image appears smooth, as if drawn by the stroke of a pen (Fig. 2.29). This appearance may be modified by: (1) poor quality of the barium film: too pale, too dense, or heterogeneous due to cracking or flocculation; (2) the presence of fecal residue, mucus, or bubbles, resulting in false images; and (3) normal elements in mucosal relief.

2.3.1 Poor Coating Quality in Double Contrast

Poor quality of the coating may have different causes:

Density Too Low. This is due to film overexposure or overdilution of the barium when water remains in the colon due to diarrhea caused by the preparation or insufficient evacuation of the cleansing enema. The contrast can be improved by extending the examination. "Cathartic colitis" is also implicated. When chronic laxative abuse is suspected, it is best to use a highly concentrated barium. (For example, Bret adds a 150 mg tube of barium sulfate (Microtrast, Nicholas Laboratories, 74240 Gaillard, France) to 500 ml of the Micropaque barium suspension.)

Density Too High. This is due to the film being underexposed, the barium being too dense, or overextended examination, causing excessive drying of the barium. This high density inhibits a detailed interpretation (Fig. 2.30). Cracking of the coating may follow. Clear lines appear, resulting in a net-like image (Fig. 2.31).

Flocculation. Flocculation corresponds to the formation of barium aggregates adhering to the colonic wall. They form opaque spots inside the marginal line, which is thus broken in places (Fig. 2.32). Where the line persists, however, it remains even. These barium aggregates are often large in size (Fig. 2.33). In any case, they make interpretation difficult.

In general, it is easy to differentiate between a mild degree of flocculation and the granular appearance of the mucosa seen in the initial stage of ulcerative colitis. The latter is seen in the first radiographs obtained, whereas flocculation does not occur until after colonic collapse, thus sparing the initial images. Distinguishing between flocculation and ulcerations is even easier. Ulceration causes the formation of "addition" images outside the marginal line.

Except in rare cases (colonic cleansing with medicinal preparations which precipitate the barium), flocculation never occurs early in the examination but

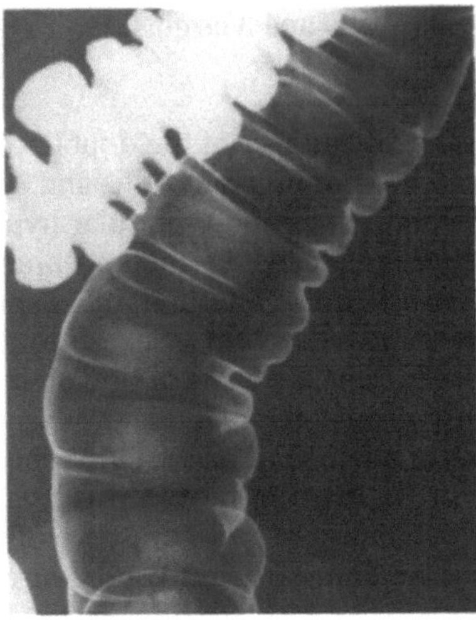

2.29

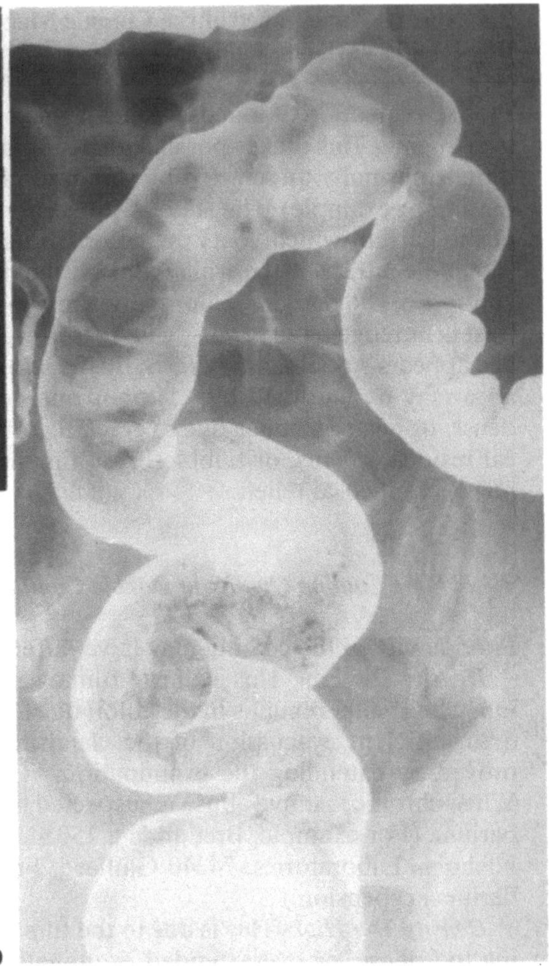

2.30

Fig. 2.29. Normal double contrast appearance

Fig. 2.30. Double contrast (too dense). The intermarginal aspect is "obscured" by the highly concentrated barium coating, or insufficiently "penetrated"

always after colonic collapse. It is favored by certain conditions: use of a high-density barium suspension, poor-quality colonic preparation, and drying of the barium coating at the end of the examination. Flocculation should and can be prevented by carrying out the examination reasonably quickly and especially by avoiding any lasting collapse during the examination. Any drainage of barium may cause collapse and should immediately be compensated for by reinjecting an equal volume of air. Collapse can also be prevented by turning the patient according to the segments to be filled by air.

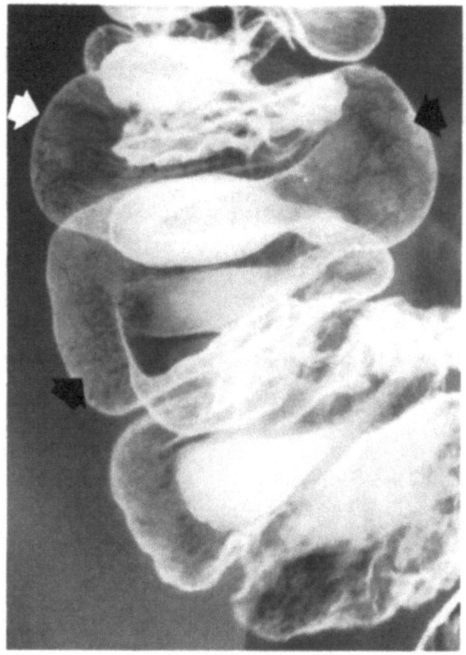

Fig. 2.31. Cracking of the barium coating *(arrows)* in the cecum at the end of the examination

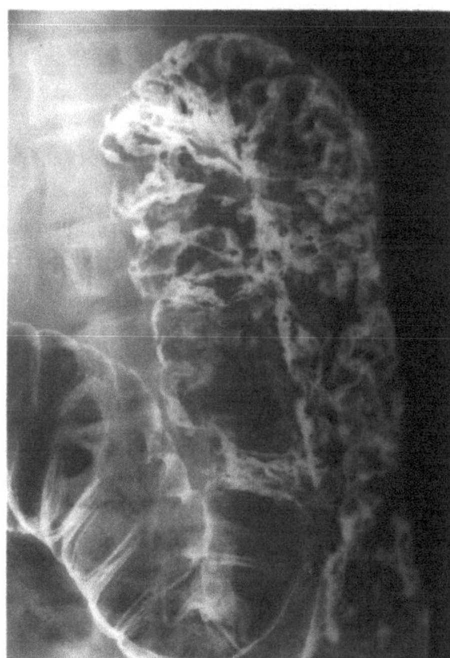

Fig. 2.33. Severe flocculation

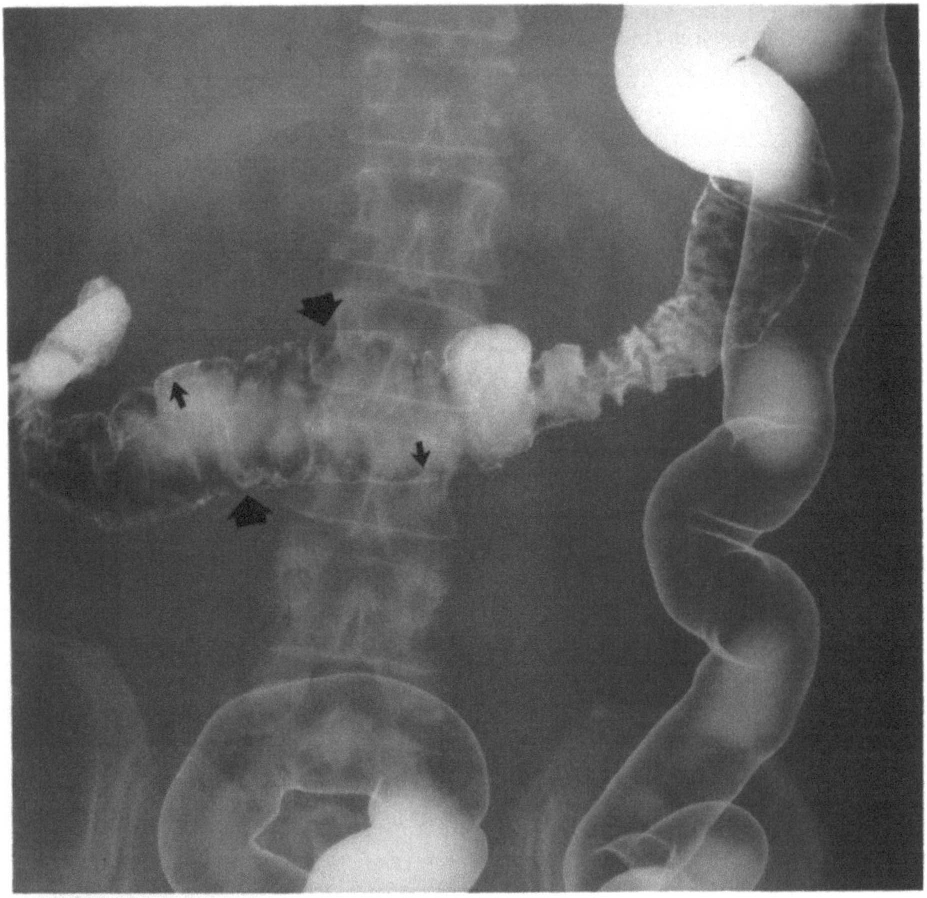

Fig. 2.32. Flocculation in the transverse colon following a spasm. Left colon: the double contrast image is normal. Transverse colon: the mucosa coating is altered in places *(large arrows)* and barium aggregates are seen in the lumen *(small arrows)*

2.3.2 *False Images*

Semiliquid fecal matter may coat the mucosa, rendering it largely heterogeneous (Fig. 2.34). A repeat examination is necessary if this happens. Major fecal stasis is rarely a problem since it should be discovered in the plain abdominal radiograph. A small quantity of adherent fecal residue will be discussed in Chap. 3. It is a problem only when there is a large amount. Colonic mucus may have several different appearances: (1) mucus strands covering an entire colonic segment which appear dense in double contrast; in a pool, they have a lacunar, stringy, combed appearance (Fig. 2.35); (2) strands or dense aggregates strung between two valves (Fig. 2.36) or with one free end in the lumen; (3) strands adhering to the wall and thus breaking the mucosal image (Fig. 2.37).

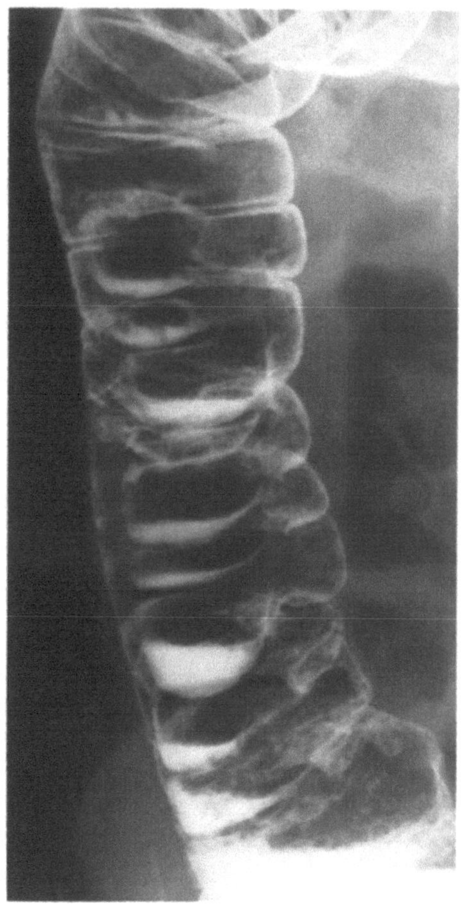

Fig. 2.34. Inadequate preparation of the cecum and ascending colon. Appearance of the colonic mucosa is highly heterogeneous; interpretation is impossible

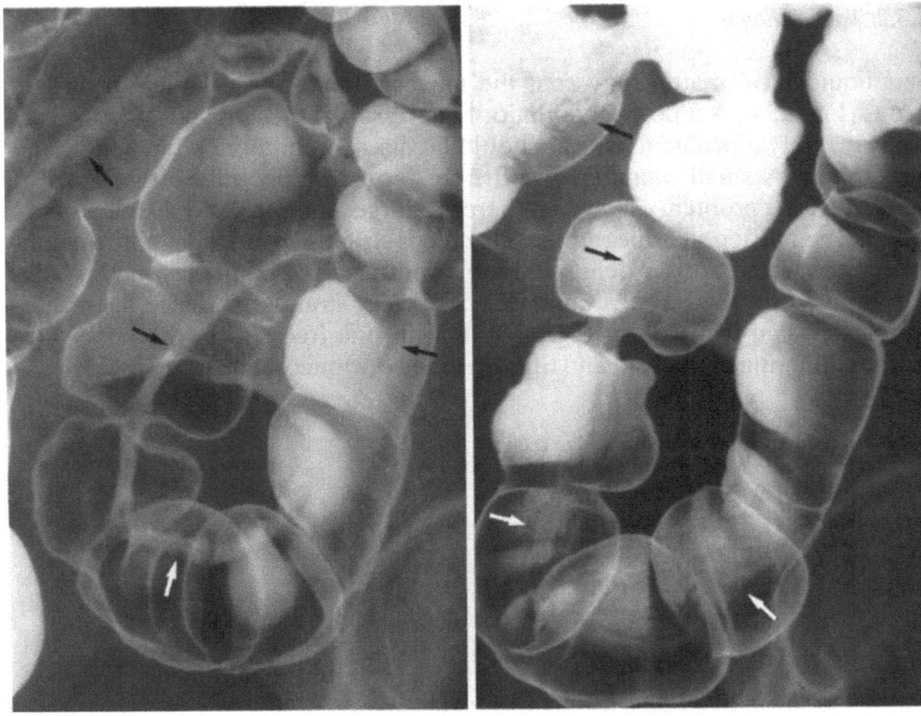

A B

Fig. 2.35. Double contrast image of a mucus strand **(A)**. In a pool **(B)** it has a lacunar, stringy, combed appearance

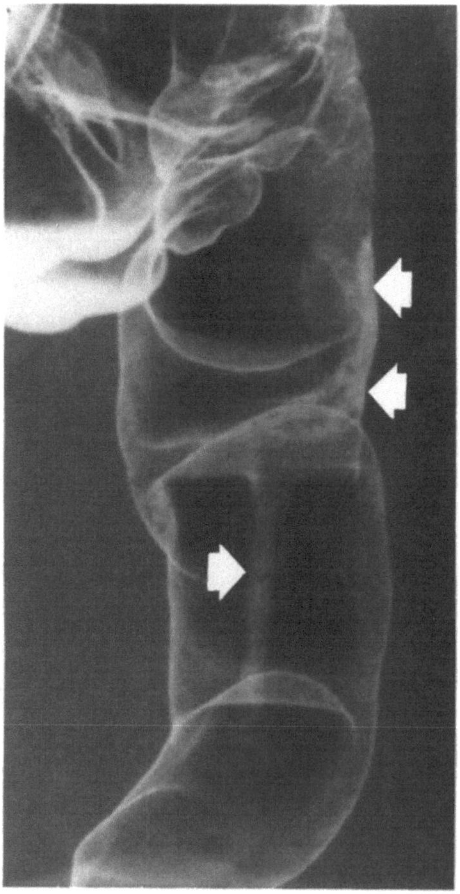

2.36

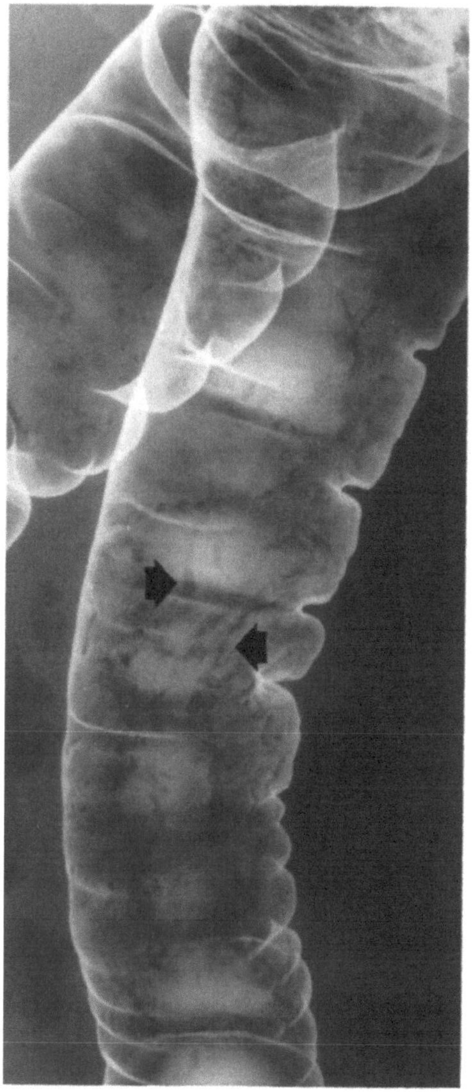

2.37

Fig. 2.36. Mucus aggregate against the wall and strung between two valves *(arrows)*

Fig. 2.37. Stringy mucus adhering to the wall with a filling defect in the pool

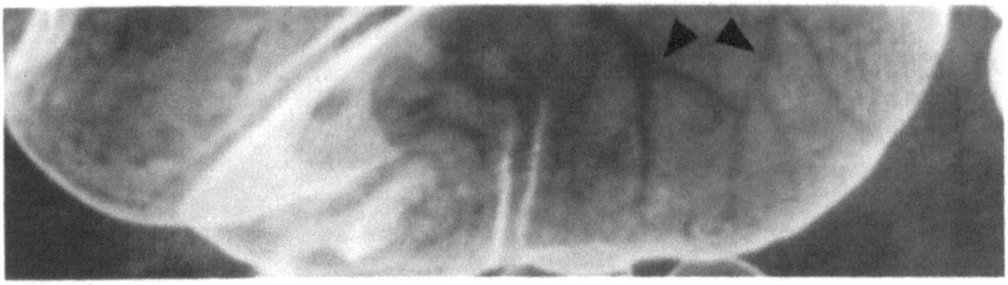

Fig. 2.38. Submucous vessels in the cecum *(arrows)*

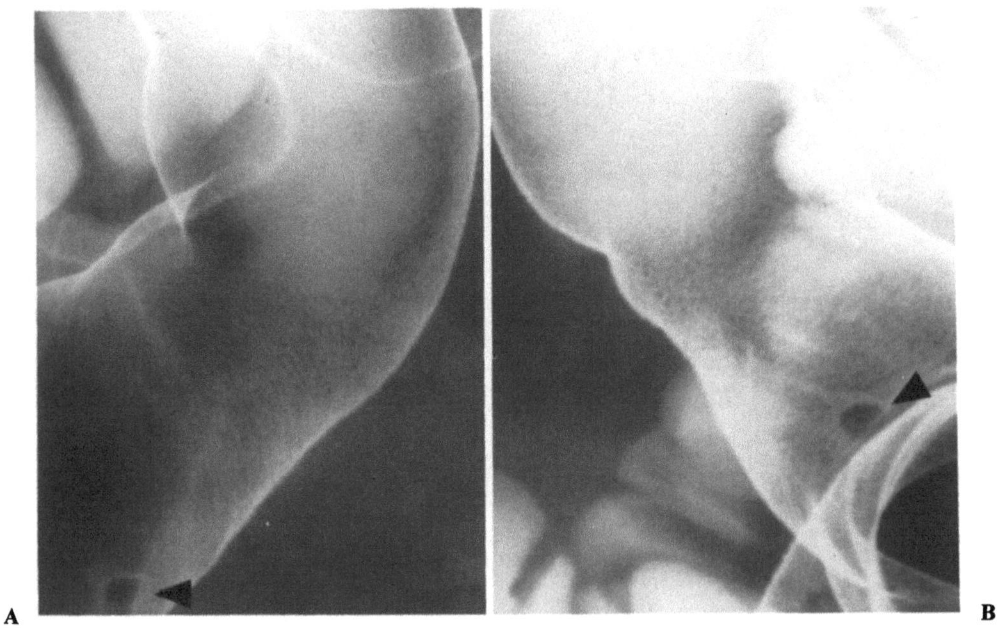

Fig. 2.39. Innominate lines: striated **(A)** and grid appearance **(B)** in the same patient. The mucosal line is broken by a sessile polyp *(arrow)*

2.3.3 Normal Modifications in the Mucosal Line

A number of normal elements in the mucosal line may modify the frontal and profile appearance of the colonic mucosa. These are: submucous vessels, innominate lines, and possibly crypts of Lieberkühn.

2.3.3.1 Submucous Vessels

Submucous vessels can be recognized by their branching (Fig. 2.38) and are rarely seen in double contrast. They correspond to the vessels seen in endoscopy.

2.3.3.2 Innominate Lines

Innominate lines are fine depressions in the colonic mucosa 0.5–2 mm apart. Three patterns have been described [7–10]: (1) linear (Fig. 2.39), where the lines, which are largely parallel, are arranged in a circular pattern and only intersect at wide intervals (striated appearance); (2) network (Figs. 2.39 B, 2.41), in which the lines form a network of meshes (grid appearance) separating sections of the colonic mucosa; and (3) mixed, in which both linear and network are combined (mixed appearance).

According to Cole [2], innominate lines are secondary to lymphoid nodules in the muscularis mucosae whose positioning exactly matches that of the lines. For some authors [7] the demonstration of innominate lines is a criterion of quality. However, the type of barium used, degree of distension, and quality of the preparation are determining factors. With the technique and barium we use, innominate lines are rarely demonstrated. They are certainly not pathologic unless possibly if highly conspicuous. Any accentuation suggests submucosal edema (Fig. 2.40) and calls for endoscopic examination and biopsy.

2.3.3.3 Physiologic Microspiculation (Pinpoint Appearance)

Physiologic microspiculation is frequent and should be recognized. For some authors, it corresponds to opacification of the crypts of Lieberkühn [3–8], and for others it corresponds to the intersection of innominate lines (Figs. 2.42, 2.43). It is seen most frequently in the rectum but may be found in any colonic segment. It is not constantly present during the examination and most often follows a spasm. It occurs in particularly well-prepared patients and corresponds to pinpoint collections of barium covering the colonic mucosa of the walls. These collections are more or less regularly distributed and, unlike aphthoid ulcers, are not surrounded by edema. In other respects, the appearance of the colonic mucosa is normal as opposed to what would be expected with ulcerative colitis. In profile, fine spiculation is seen which, in general, does not exceed 1 mm in depth. It appears and is particularly visible with partial distension and disappears with total distension (Fig. 2.41). In our experience, physiologic microspiculation is quite different from that observed in the early stages of colitis (Crohn's disease and ulcerative colitis). A high degree of spiculation may, however, call for endoscopic examination (Fig. 2.43).

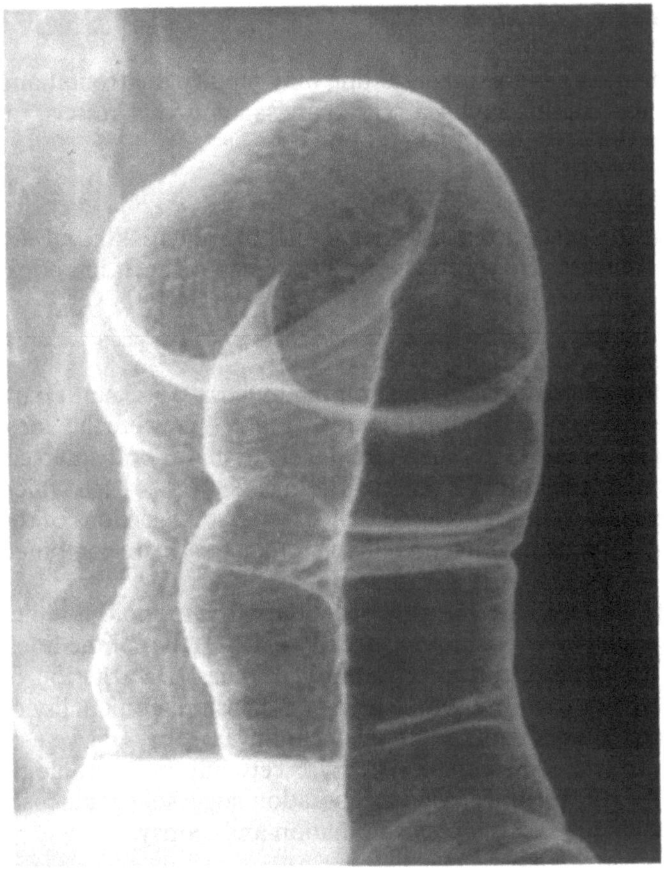

Fig. 2.40. Abnormal accentuation of innominate lines (operated Crohn's disease, right hemicolectomy). Biopsy, severe chorionic edema

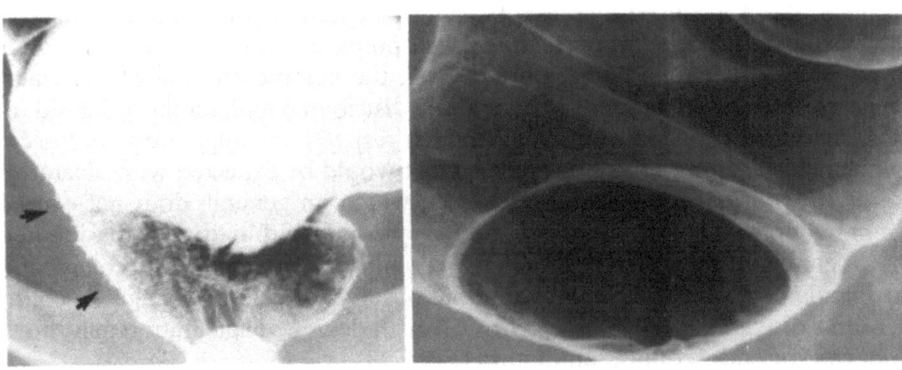

A B

Fig. 2.41. A, grid and pinpoint appearance with microspiculation of the margins *(arrows)*; B, disappearance of this image with total distention

A

B

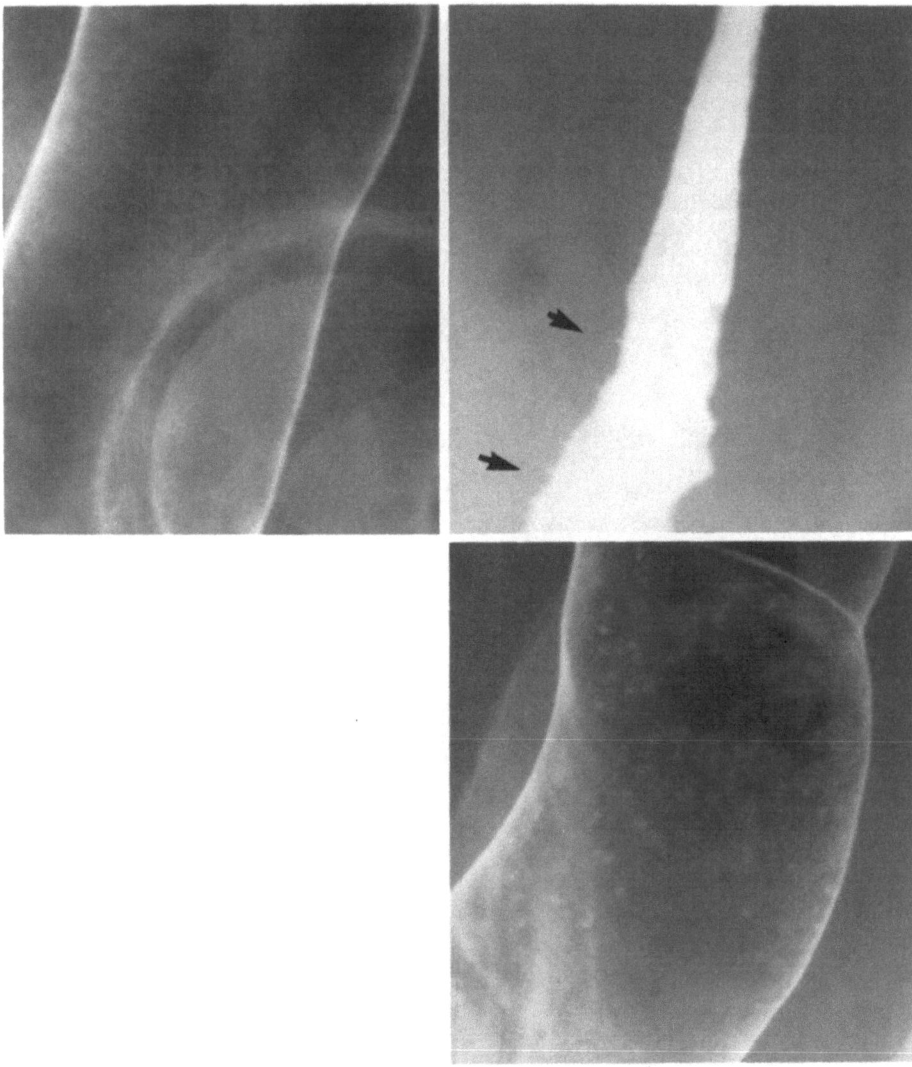

C

Fig. 2.42. A, Normal appearance. **B** Spasm with microspiculation of the margins *(arrows)*. **C** marginal spiculation disappears but the pinpoint appearance of the wall remains after distention

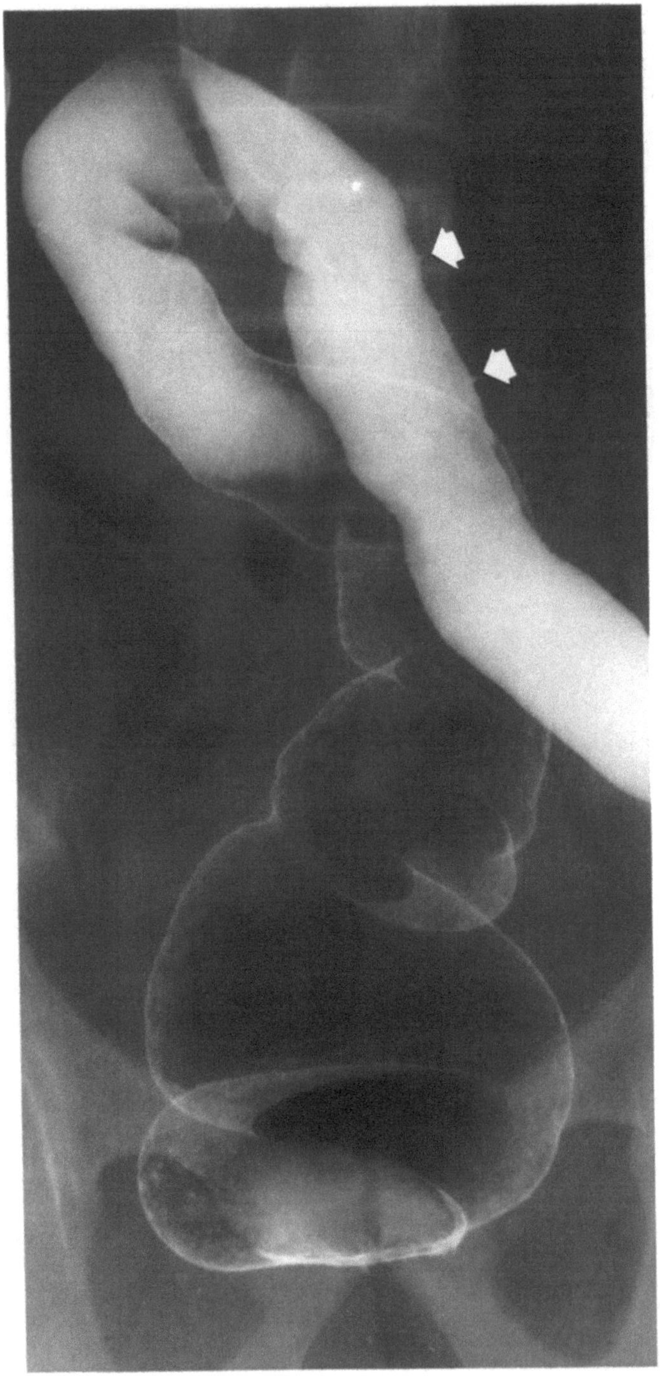

Fig. 2.43. Pronounced spiculation of the sigmoid *(arrows)* and rectum *(pinpoint appearance)*. While probably not pathologic, such an image may require endoscopic verification

2.4 Interpreting the Examination

A thorough study must be made. The technique we recommend to our students is as follows:

1. The radiographs are displayed before the patient leaves the examination room on a screen large enough to show, if not all the radiographs, at least all those concerning a particular colonic segment.

2. The quality of the preparation is evaluated; it is considered excellent when no fecal residue is visible, good when some is visible but does not interfere (little free residue), or poor when there is much residue and it is adherent or if there is scybala or fluid fecal matter coating the mucosa, making the double contrast heterogeneous. If it is only at his stage that the preparation is judged to be poor, any satisfactory interpretation is impossible. The examination should be repeated under better conditions.

3. The morphology of the colon (position and length) is considered.

4. The segments are analyzed, one by one: rectum - sigmoid - iliac - descending - splenic flexure - transverse - hepatic flexure - ascending - cecum. Each segment, insufflated or not, should be analyzed in each radiograph as it appears. For each segment, the study includes: the caliber, appearance of the haustra, appearance of the colonic mucosa: frontal and in profil, appearance of any pools which are present, and filling defects or other elementary images. This study should be carried out very carefully and thoroughly.

5. Results of the examination should include: the type of preparation used (and any medicinal hypotonia reported), motor activity results obtained during filling and a description of any problems that might have occurred, whether insufflation was painful or not, an evaluation of the quality of the preparation, and the actual report of the examination.

References

1. Bret P (1981) Radiologie de l'intestin grêle et du côlon. SIMEP (38-46 rue de bruxelles - Villeurbane - France) pp 68-73
2. Cole P (1978) Innominate grooves of the colon: the morphological characteristics and etiologic mechanisms. Radiology 128: 41-43
3. Dassel PM (1962) Innocuous filling of the intestinal glands of the colon during barium enema (spiculation) simulating organic disease. Radiology 78: 799-801
4. Davenport HW (1976) Physiologie de l'appareil digestif. Masson, Paris
5. Farrar CW (1979) Patterns of sigmoïd colon and their implications for barium enema radiography. Medical Radiography and Photography 5: 2-28
6. Marshak RH (1975) Granulomatous disease of the intestinal tract. Radiology 114: 3-32
7. Matsuura K, Nakata H, Takeda N, Nakata S, Shimoda Y (1977) Innominate lines of the colon. Radiological histological correlation. Radiology 125: 571-584
8. Sasson L, Bronx NY (1960) Entrance of barium into intestinal glands during barium enema. JAMA 173: 343-345
9. Weissman A, Bousquet JC, Harriague D, Grellet J (1980) Aspects de l'anatomie radiologique du côlon en double contraste. J Radiol Electrol 61: 301-311
10. Williams I (1965) Innominate grooves in the surface mucosa. Radiology 84: 877-880
11. Wolf S (1976) Physiology of the colon. In: Bockus HL (ed) Gastroenterology T III, Saunders, London pp 803-815

3 Radiologic Signs in Tumoral Pathology: Polyps and Polyposis Syndromes

3.1 Introduction

The radiologic appearance of tumors in double contrast is quite different from that observed in standard radiology. Whereas in standard radiology, stenosis and filling defects represent the radiologic signs of tumors, double contrast images are more complex and include three types:

1. Tumoral contour images by the tangent effect (polycyclic or circle images); by accumulation of barium at the base of a lesion (Welin's "bowler hat sign") or in tumoral irregularities; and by appearance of the tumor in a barium pool (filling defect)

2. Tumoral surface images by the additon effect: overlapping of barium coatings of the tumor and colonic walls ("hat sign," addition image)

3. Colonic contour changes caused by the tumor (stenosis, indentation) If filling defects are to be included with these signs, they are less important. With the single contrast technique, the larger the lesion, the more clearly it appears. In double contrast, size does not play as important a role. It is by analysis of all the linear images and filling defects, to determine whether or not they correspond to normal anatomic structures by their form and position, that leads to the detection of abnormal images. One of the major principles in interpreting double contrast is the careful analysis of images and their reasoned interpretation. Since not all images have a corresponding logical explanation (anatomic or artifact), they should be considered pathologic until proven otherwise. While advanced tumors may be more difficult to detect for the nonexperienced observer, they do have different but obvious radiologic signs when the quality of the examination is good and its interpretation thorough.

3.2 Polyps

The major (but not the only) interest of double contrast is in detecting polyps. A number of facts demonstrate the importance of this detection.

1. It is now largely agreed that glandular polyps are the origin of rectocolic cancer. (The term polyp here has only a macroscopic definition: "small growth on the colonic mucosa" and does not take into consideration the histologic nature of the lesion.)

2. The 5-year survival rate for operated rectocolic cancers is between 50% and 60%. This rate has not increased despite surgical progress, whereas the

5-year survival rate for cancer discovered in the early stage is greater than 90%.

3. Destruction of all polyps discovered through routine rectoscopy reduces the incidence of rectal cancer by 85% [5].

These facts show that, while the chances of increasing the survival rate for patients with rectocolic cancer are few, prevention is possible by detecting polyps. The question of asymptomatic patients remains unanswered (chemical test for fecal occult blood or flexible fiberoptic proctosigmoidoscopy as a routine diagnostic procedure?). When examination of the colon is requested by the internist, double contrast seems to be the examination of choice. It provides for a complete examination under conditions often much less uncomfortable than those of colonoscopy. In particular, it provides for a reliable examination of the colon as opposed to the standard barium enema which, according to Williams et al. [19], leaves 82% of polyps less than 1 cm and 22% more than 1 cm undetected. These values are 23% and 2% respectively for double contrast.

Some time ago, Welin et al. [17] established that the level of polyp detection for patients examined by double contrast varies between 10% and 13%; a level which approaches that of discovery during autopsy. This corresponds to approximately the same level for all radiologic departments using double contrast in Europe and the United States, whereas the level of polyp detection for the standard technique remains fixed at between 1% and 4% (rarely 8%). In light of this, *the double contrast barium enema should, except where contraindicated, replace the traditional barium enema.*

3.2.1 Macroscopic Appearance of Polyps

Three different macroscopic types of polyp, each having its own radiologic appearance, should be distinguished:

1. The *sessile* polyp appears as a tumor whose base is its largest part. It may be flat like a watch crystal.
2. The *intermediate* polyp narrows at its parietal implantation, thus creating a recess where barium may penetrate. This appearance seen through endoscopy seems to precede stalk formation. A stalk may form temporarily during endoscopic examination by traction exerted on the tumor. It is thus quite short.
3. The *pedunculated* polyp is clearly differentiated from the wall to which it is joined by a stalk variable in size and form. The stalk is formed by traction exerted by the polyp on the colonic mucosa during passage of the fecal bolus.

3.2.2 Radiologic Polyp Images

3.2.2.1 Sessile Polyps

The sessile polyp has three radiologic images depending on whether it is seen frontally, from a three-quarter view, or in profile (Figs. 3.1, 3.2).

Frontally, the image is a *dense circle* outlining the tumoral contour *(ring shadow).* The image is most often clear and regular. Its form is usually round but may be oval or polycyclic. Density of the field inside the circle is less than or

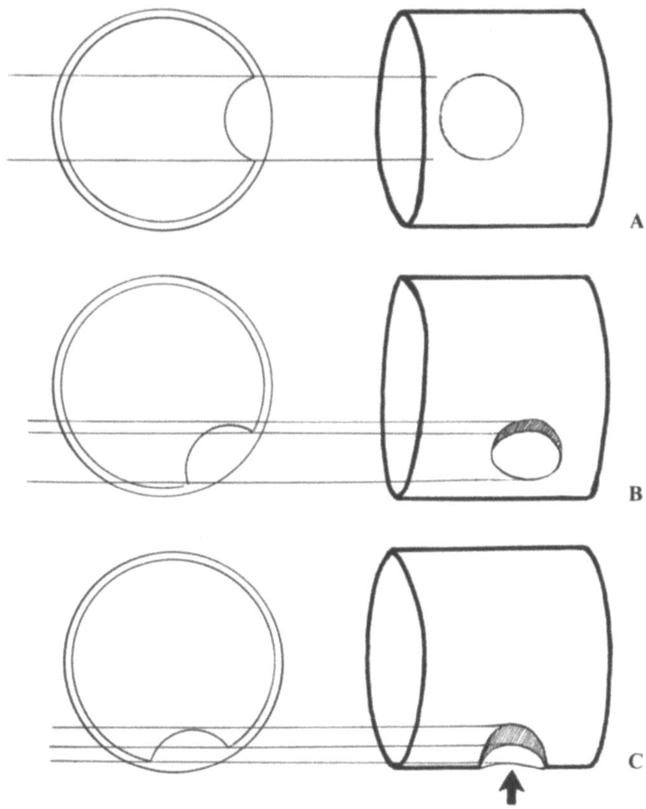

Fig. 3.1. Diagrammatic representation of the formation of a sessile polyp image: **A,** frontal: ring shadow; **B,** three-quarter view: hat sign (addition effect); **C,** profile (it is not a strict profile in this diagram): an indentation is seen at the base of the lesion *(arrow)*

equal to that of the adjacent wall. Only in rare cases does a barium droplet on the polyp dome increase the density at the center of the image (stalactite image).

From a three-quarter view, the base of the lesion is indicated by a circle or oval which is more or less complete depending on the slope of the incident beam. If the polyp is sufficiently raised, a dense crescent image formed by the four overlapping barium layers covering the polyp and bowel wall will cap the circle of the base (Fig. 3.1-3.4). This is what we call the *"hat sign",*[1] which has an important diagnostic value since it does not seem to appear for air bubbles and rarely for fecal matter. Disappearance of a segment of the circle marking the base of the lesion is possible *(erasure sign).* This disappearance is located on the side opposite the "hat." It occurs when the incident beam is no longer tangent to the curve joining the polyp to the wall (Figs. 3.5, 3.6).

---

1 Welin' "bowler hat" sign is slightly different (see Sect. 3.2.2.2).

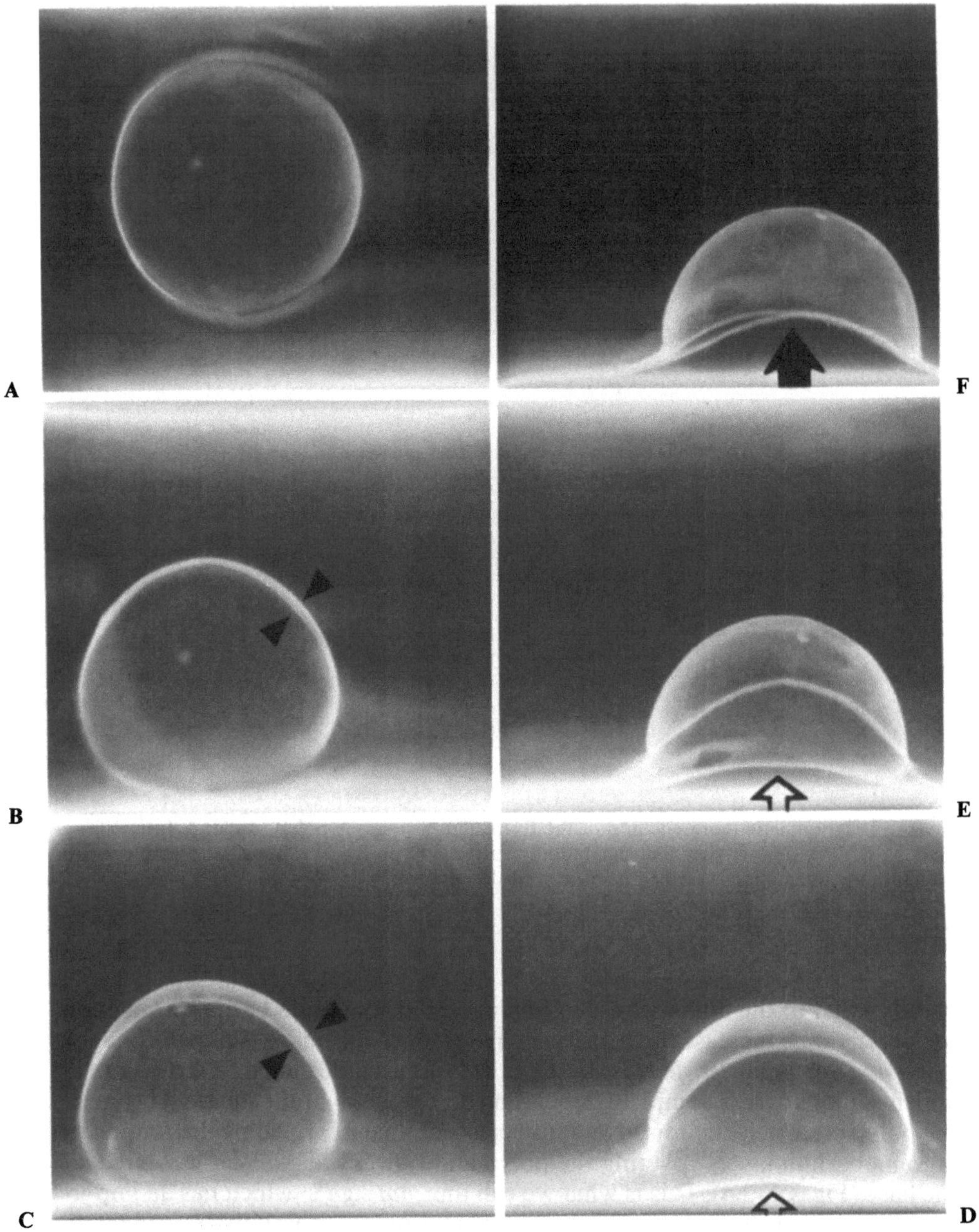

Fig. 3.2. Simulation montage of a sessile polyp: (plastic hemisphere attached to the inside of a jelly jar). **A,** frontal: Ring shadow; **B, C,** three-quarter view: appearance of hat sign *(arrows)* and disappearance of the opposite border; **D, E,** more pronounced three-quarter view: indentation *(arrow)*; **F,** the indentation *(arrow)* and polyp dome are easily seen in strict profile

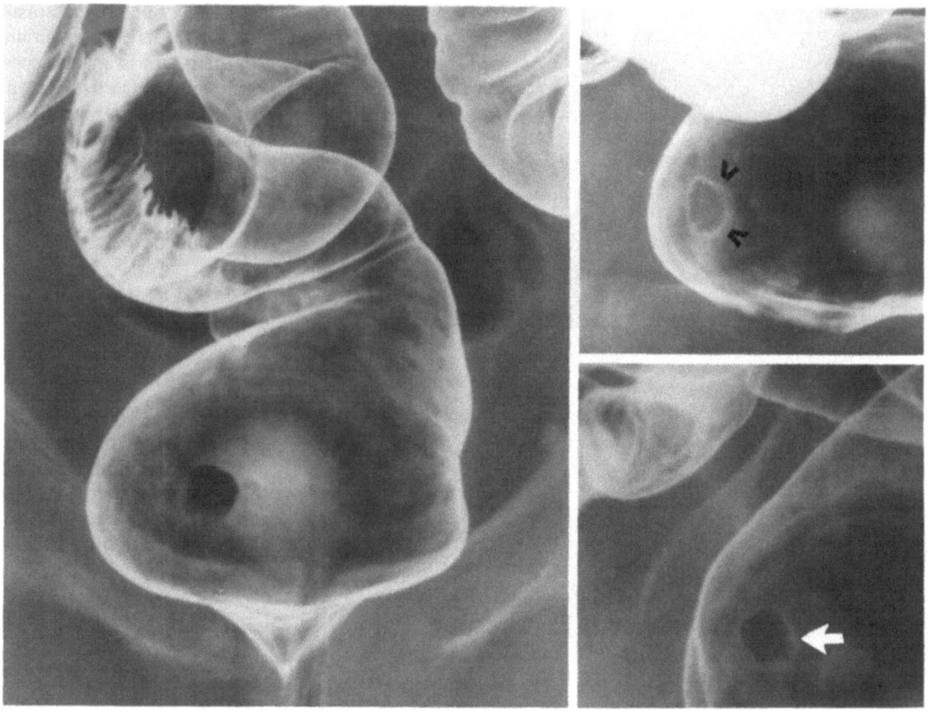

A B C

Fig. 3.3. Rectal sessile polyp (benign): **A,** filling defect in a pool (frontal); **B,** a slight hat sign appears (three-quarter view); **C,** ring shadow (frontal)

Fig. 3.4. Sessile polyp (adenocarcinoma) (the polyp is projected on the femoral head below the articulation). Hat sign: **a,** base ring shadow; **b,** polyp dome (hat)

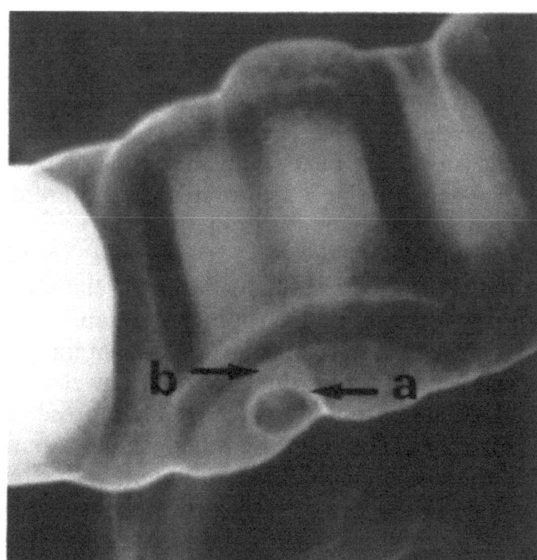

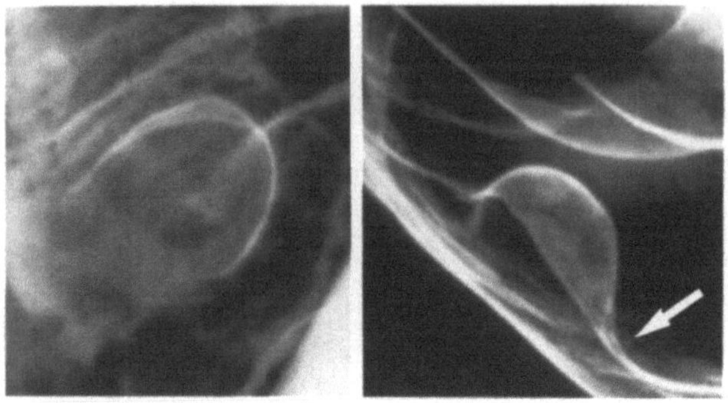

Fig. 3.5. Sessile polyp. Erasure sign: **On the left,** the lower limit of the tumor is erased (cecal sessile polyp). **On the right,** a radiograph taken in profile shows the junction between the polyp and the wall. In the frontal radiograph, the incident beam was not tangent to this curved junction

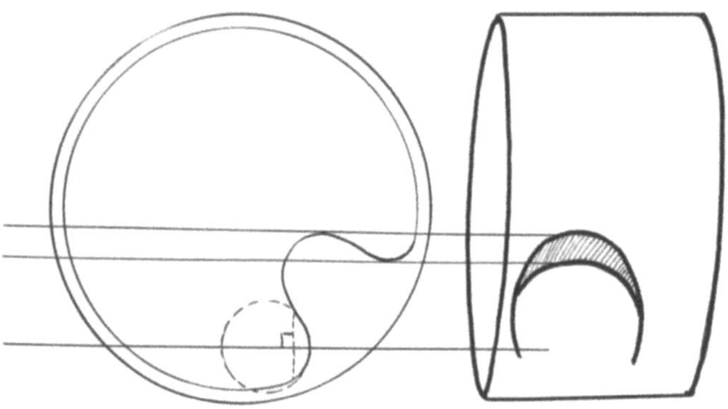

Fig. 3.6. Sessile polyp. Erasure sign: the incident beam is no longer tangent to the curve joining the polyp to the wall. Part of the base ring shadow is erased

In profile, we observe the formation of a dense, usually hemispheric, image due to the overlapping of four barium coatings (two of the bowel walls and two of the polyp walls; Figs. 3.1, 3.7). The image has a distinct limit toward the lumen (due to the beam tangent to the polyp dome). Its base is variable in appearance depending on the polyp's circumferential spread and the curvature of the segment on which it is implanted.

Variations in the Base Appearance According to the Polyp's Circumferential Spread. If the base of the polyp is relatively narrow, it does not separate from the bowel wall image (points A, B, and C in Fig. 3.8 a are practically aligned). However, when the lesion spreads laterally (circumferentially), the limits of its base separate from the "normal" bowel wall image (points A and B are clearly dissociated from point C, which represents the theoretical site of the wall) (Fig. 3.8 b). The resulting image shows a parietal cut or indentation at the base of the lesion (Fig. 3.9). Consequently, this indicates the size of the tumoral implantation and in no way indicates the extent of its penetration.

Variations in the Base Appearance According to the Caliber of the Colonic Segment on Which the Polyp is Implanted (Fig. 3.10). A look at Fig. 3.10 makes it easy to understand how a lesion of a given size may cause an indentation on a small-diameter segment and none on a larger-caliber segment. Another group confirmed this interpretation and used an algebraic equation to express the degree of indentation of the lesions's base [1].

The appearance of the polyp base varies according to the incidence of the beam with respect to the axis of the colonic segment in question. If there is a parietal indentation and if the incident beam is not perpendicular to the colonic axis, a helical image may form (Fig. 3.11).

Flat Polyps. Certain extremely flat (watch crystal) polyps are represented only by a ring shadow (Fig. 3.12). More infrequently they form a parietal notch (plateau image; Fig. 3.13) seen in strict profile, which is difficult to obtain. In these cases, the hat sign is not always present and sometimes reduced to a simple reinforcement of one of the margins of the ring shadow.

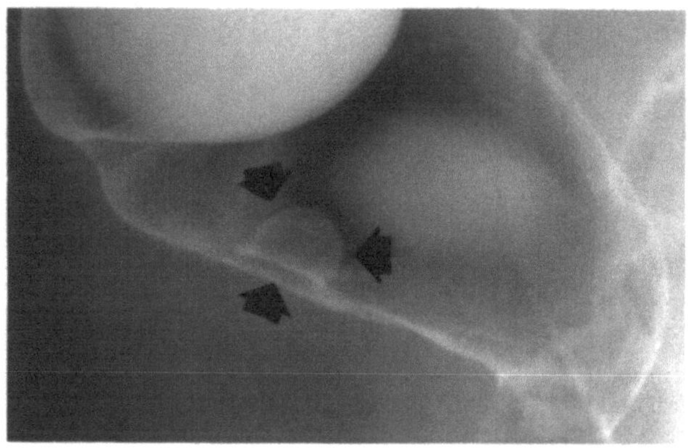

Fig. 3.7. Profile view of a sessile polyp *(arrows):* The tumor dome is dense and clearly outlined. There is no indentation in the base

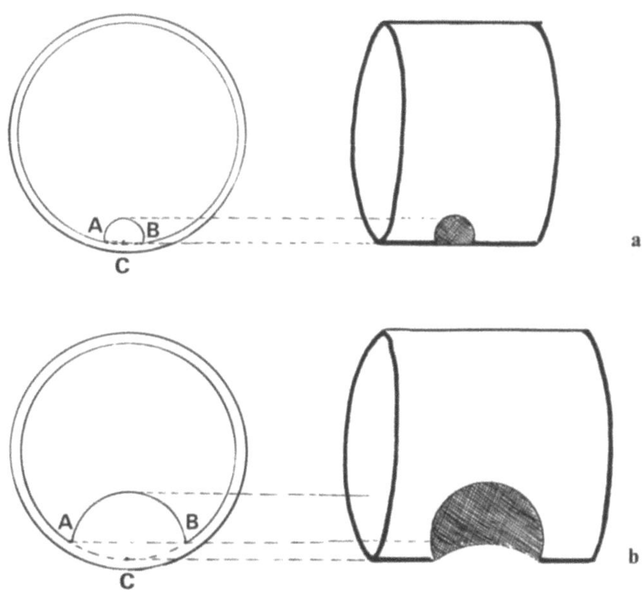

Fig. 3.8. Appearance of the base of a sessile lesion: **a,** narrow-base lesion: points **A** and **B** (junction points between the polyp and colonic wall) do not separate from point **C,** which is the theoretical site of the wall. **b,** wide-base lesion: points **A** and **B** rise and clearly separate from point **C.** The result is an indentation image

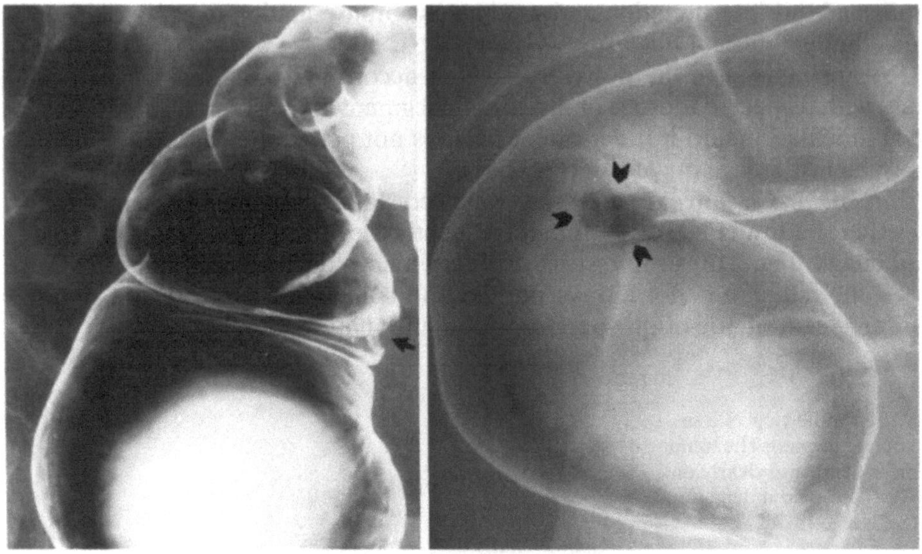

A B

Fig. 3.9. **A** Profile view of a villoma shows an indentation at the base of the lesion *(arrow)*. **B** The lesion appears frontally in a radiograph taken in profile *(arrows)*. It has a large base, which explains the indentation

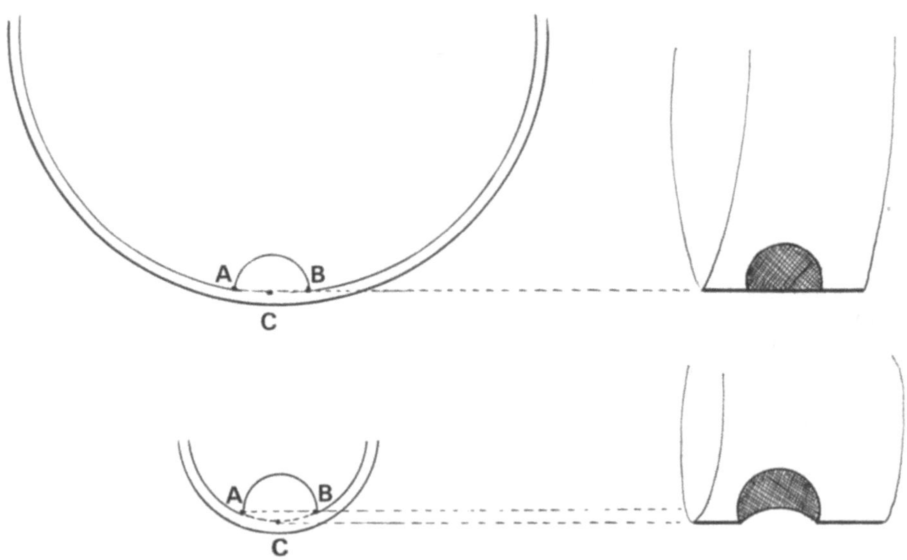

Fig. 3.10. Appearance of the base of a sessile polyp: for the same size base, an indentation appears only of the segment smaller radius

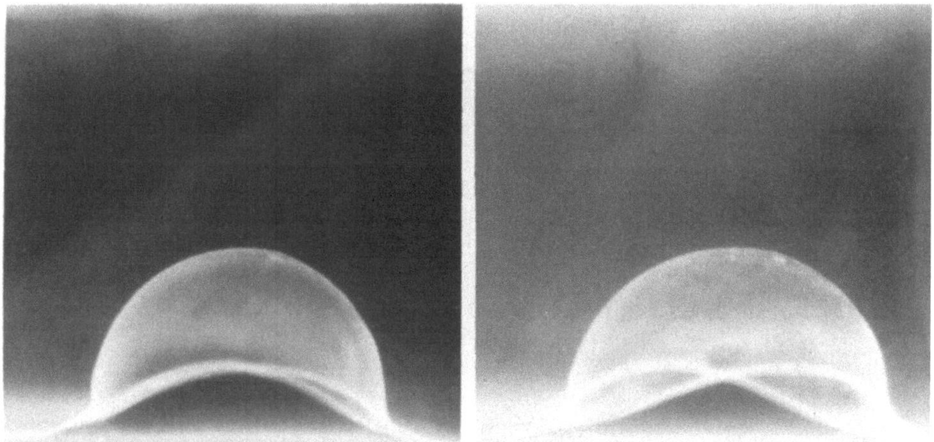

A B

Fig. 3.11. Appearance of the base according to the incident angle (montage): **A** The incident beam is perpendicular to the axis of the colonic segment containing the tumor. The base of the lesion is clearly seen since the lesion is in strict profile. **B** The incident beam is no longer perpendicular to the axis of the colonic segment. The resulting image of the base is helical and the indentation is not as distinct

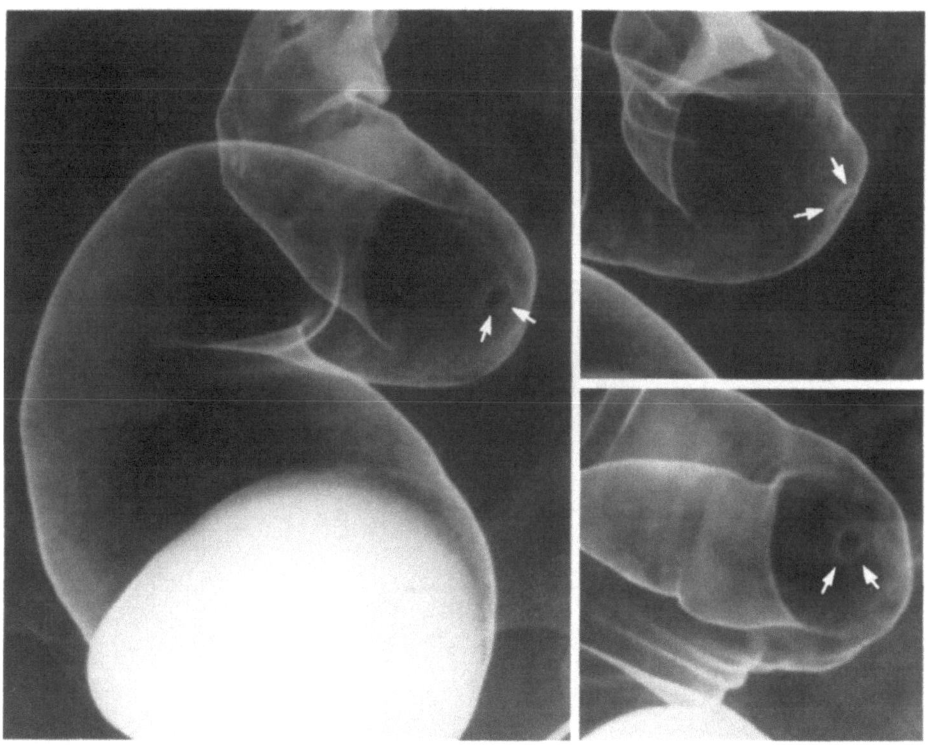

A B C

Fig. 3.12. Sessile micropolyp (flat): **A,** three-quarter view: oval image *(arrow)*; **B,** frontal view: Ring shadow *(arrow)*; **C,** more pronounced three-quarter view: minimal hat sign *(arrows)*

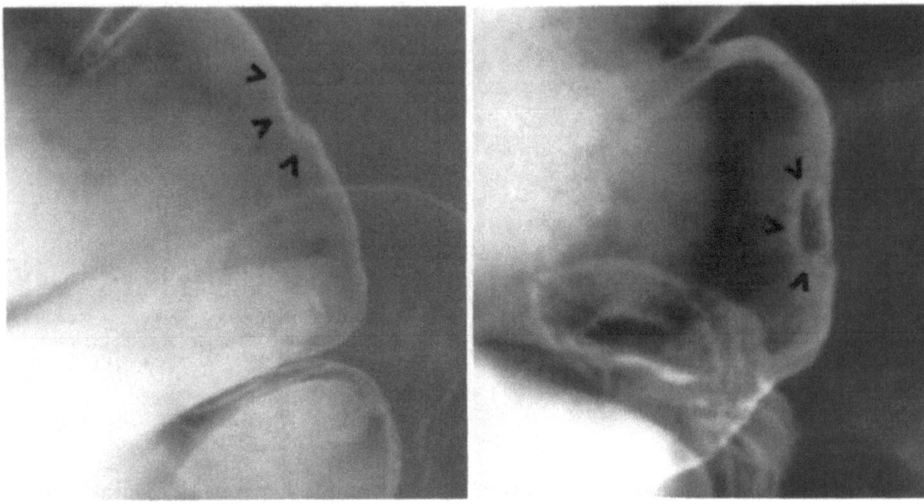

A B

Fig. 3.13. Plateau polyp: A, minimal parietal notch; B, ring shadow without hat sign

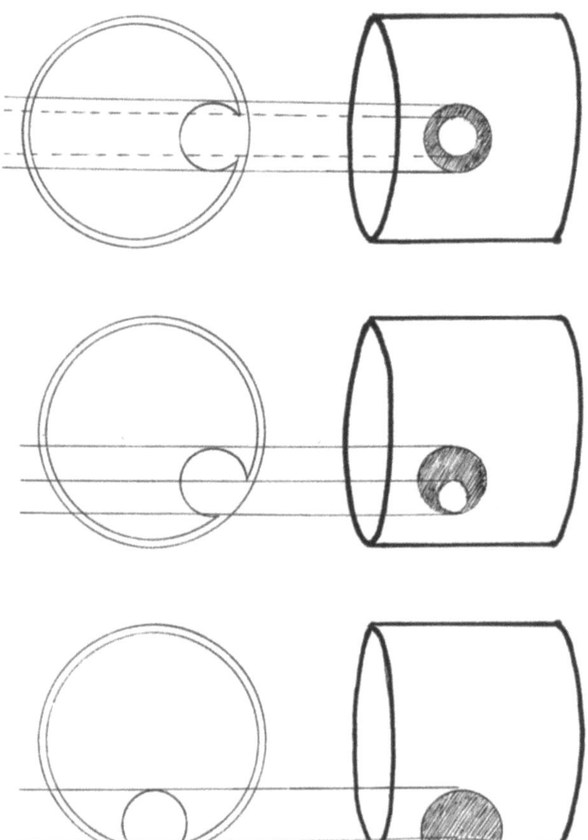

Fig. 3.14. Diagrammatic representation of the formation of an intermediate polyp image: A, frontal target or ring image; B, three-quarter view hat sign; off-center target; C, profile

A

B

C

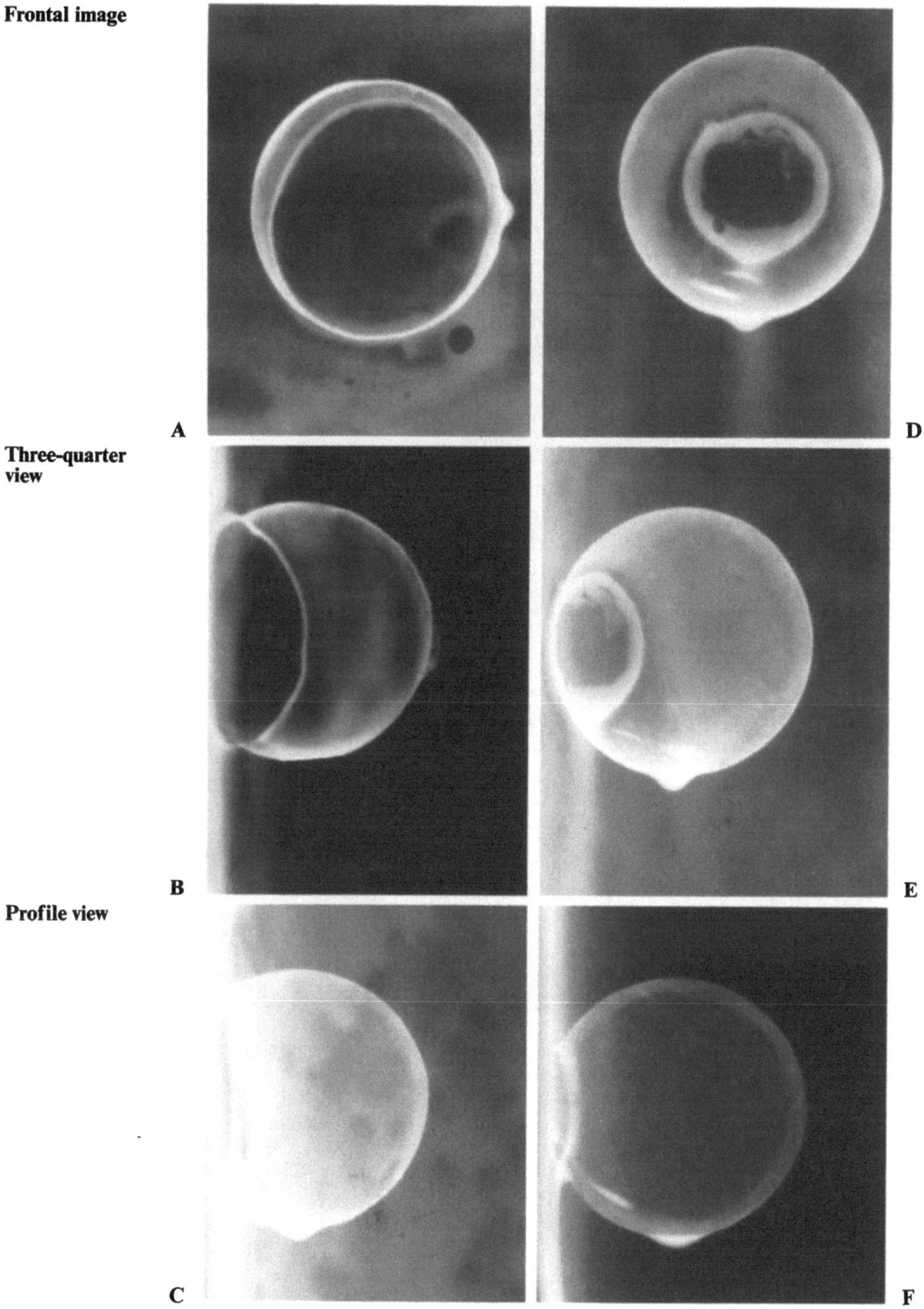

Fig. 3.15. Montage of intermediate polyps: **A, B, C,** wide-base polyp; **A,** ring image; **B,** hat sign; **C,** strict profile; **D, E, F,** narrow-base polyp; **D,** target image; **E,** off-center target; **F,** profile

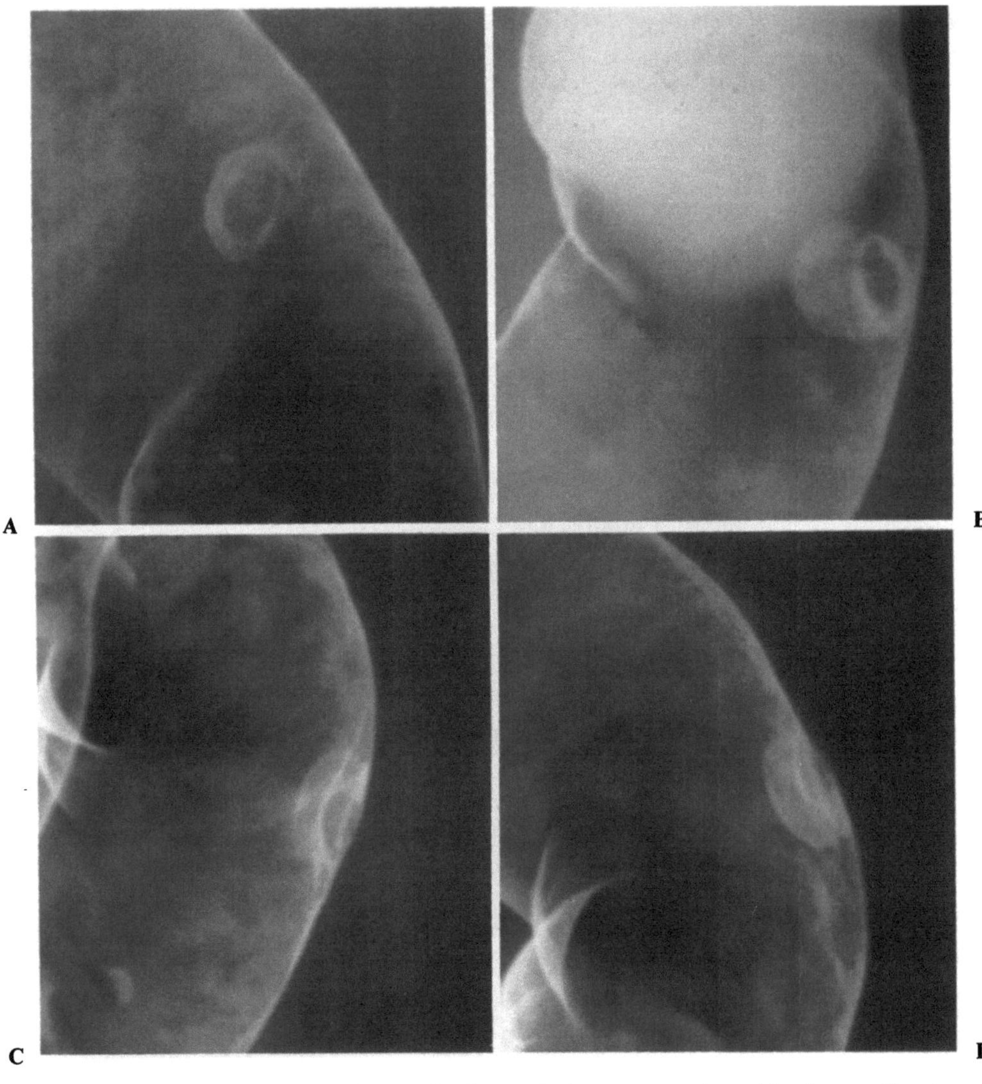

Fig. 3.16. Intermediate polyp: **A,** frontal: ring image; **B,** three-quarter view: either hat or off-center target; **C, D,** strict profile: absence of indentation

3.2.2.2 Intermediate Polyps (Figs. 3.14, 3.15)

The characteristic of intermediate polyps is the appearance of a second circled image formed by the incident beam tangent to the periphery of the polyp. Relations between this second circle and the base circle vary depending of the incidence. Between the two circles, the polyp appears denser than the adjacent wall since the incident beam crosses four barium coatings (two on the bowel walls and two on the polyp walls), whereas beams reflected from the base cross only two (one bowel wall and the polyp dome).

Frontally, a ring or target image is obtained whose clear center corresponds to the polyp base (Figs. 3.16, 3.17).

From a three-quarter view (Figs. 3.16, 3.17) the base is no longer projected in the center of the image. The result is an off-center target resembling our hat image. Accumulation of barium at the base of the lesion led Welin [17] to propose the "bowler hat" sign. In this case, the hat's rim corresponds to the thick circle of barium surrounding the polyp base and the center to the polyp dome.

In profile (Figs. 3.16, 3.17) the base appearance is related to the same laws of geometric projection as for sessile polyps; the appearance of the dome depends on the form of the polyp.

A 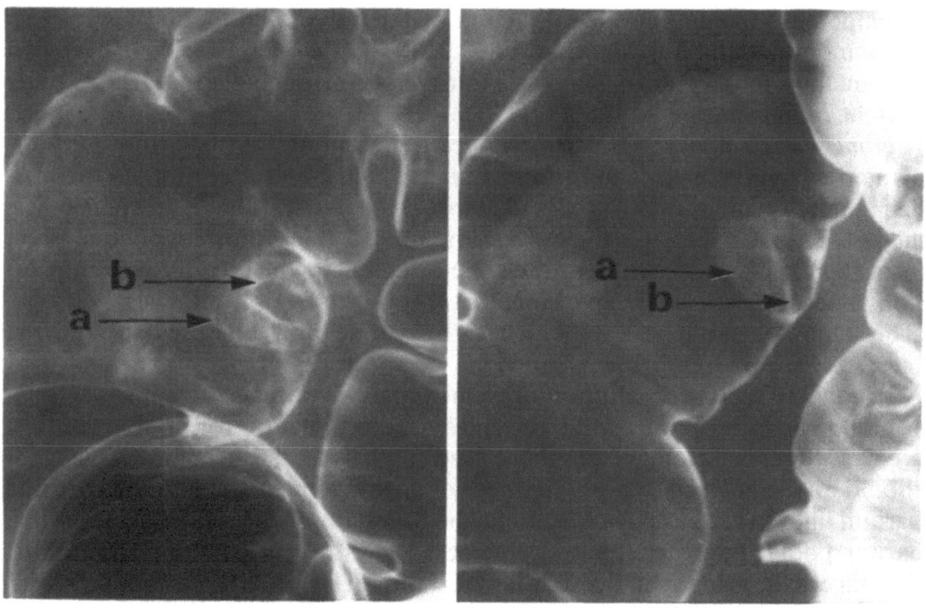 B

Fig. 3.17. Intermediate polyp: **A,** frontal; **a,** polyp dome; **b,** base image is not perfectly round (we still speak of a target image); **B,** three-quarter view: off-center target

3.2.2.3 Pedunculated Polyps (Figs. 3.18, 3.19)
A number of anatomic elements contribute to the formation of the image of pedunculated polyps: the polyp dome (represented by a circle whose interior is denser than the adjacent wall); the circle formed by the junction of the stalk and dome; the cylinder formed by the stalk; and the circle corresponding to the implantation of the stalk into the wall (when clearly individualized) (Figs. 3.18–3.20).

Frontally the image is a target whose center is lighter than the periphery and corresponds to the stalk. In this case, the incident beam is parallel to the stalk's major axis and crosses only two barium coatings (one on the bowel wall opposite the implantation and the other on the polyp dome). Adjacent beams cross both colonic walls and both aspects of the polyp. According to Welin [17], this target image is characteristic of and indicates the presence of a stalk. In our experience, this image is also obtained for narrow-based intermediate polyps. This very characteristic image should in itself draw the radiologist's attention to the probable existence of a polyp.

In profile, the stalk is clearly seen since the incident beam is perpendicular to its major axis. It is represented either by longitudinal lines which cross the transversal lines formed by haustral folds or by a filling defect (Figs. 3.21, 3.22). A temporary indentation due to traction by the polyp on the wall may form at the point of parietal implantation (Fig. 3.22 B). In the intermarginal aspect, this implantation most often appears as a transverse linear image (Fig. 3.22 B), or as a circle, or may not be visible (Fig. 3.21).

From a three-quarter view, the cylinder representing the stalk and both implantation zones combine to form an image which varies according to the incident angle. An off-center target is the most characteristic image. In some cases, the polyp dome may touch the bowel (Fig. 3.23). A thick, blurred, opaque circle forms by capillary attraction at the zone of contact, which could make the lesion appear as a sessile polyp except that this is usually only a transitory image. (The same phenomenon may occur for sessile and intermediate polyps; Figs. 3.24, 3.25.)

In concluding this description of elementary polyp images, we must emphasize one particular point: while the rules of interpretation for double contrast are considerably different from those used for the standard technique, the latter should not be neglected. A polyp does not always appear surrounded by a fine barium line. In certain positions it may be found on the dependent surface in a barium pool from which it barely emerges. Therefore, the resulting characteristic image is the same as in the standard technique: clear filling defects with definite contours in an opaque pool. This sign is of the utmost importance. It may, nevertheless, go unrecognized if one is restricted to studying clear spots and neglects the analysis of double contrast "opacities."

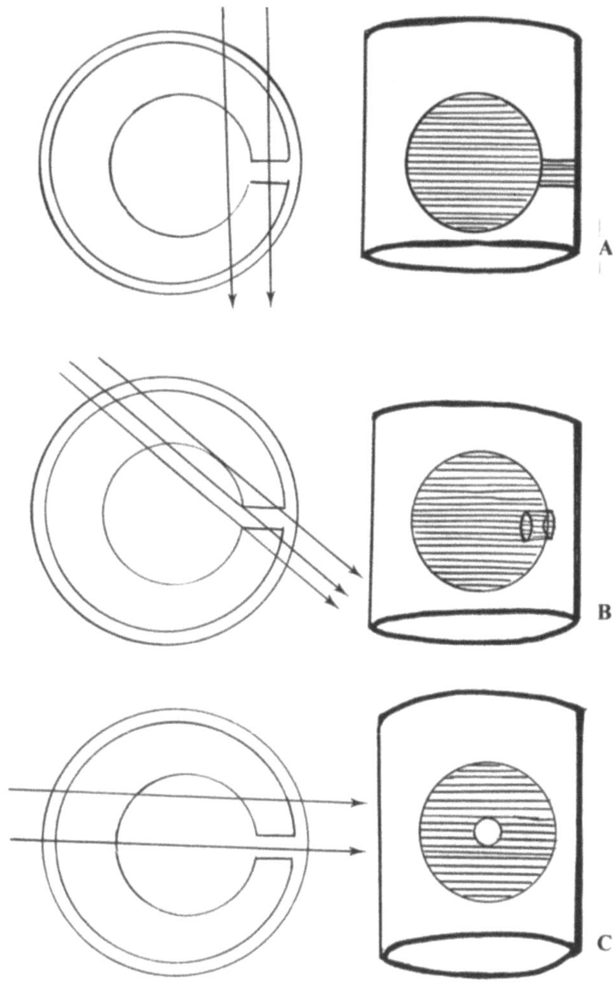

Fig. 3.18. Diagrammatic representation of the formation of a pedunculated polyp; **A,** profile: addition and tangent image; the stalk is clearly visible; **B,** three-quarter view: approaching the off-center target image; **C,** frontal view: target image

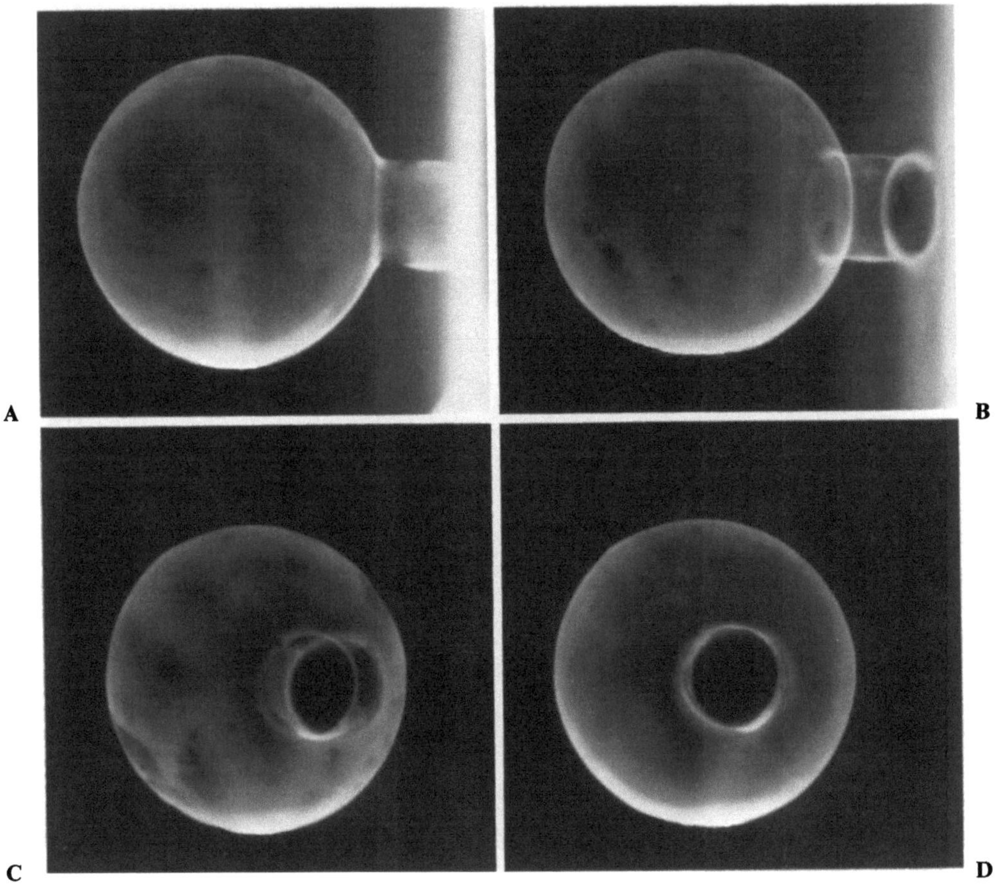

Fig. 3.19. Montage of a pedunculated polyp: **A,** profile; **B, C,** three-quarter view; **D,** frontal view

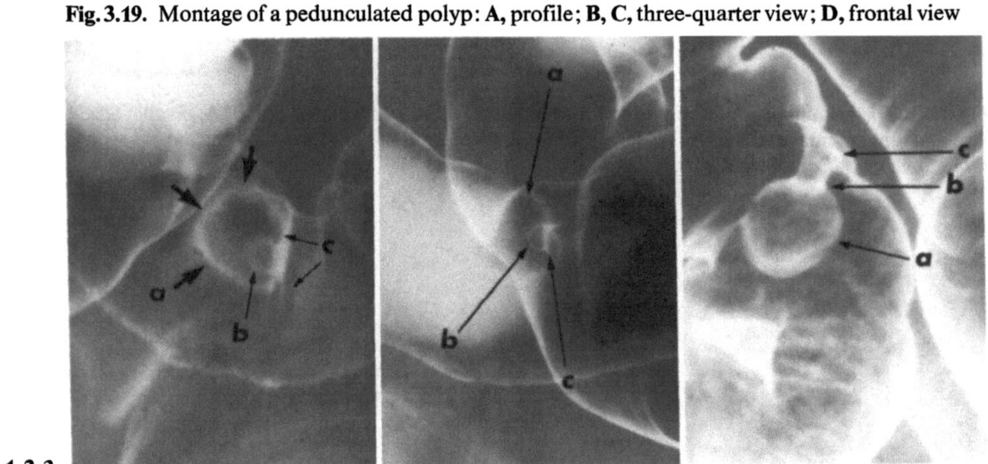

Fig. 3.20. Pedunculated polyp (villous polyadenoma); **1,** three-quarter view: off-center target; **2,** half view: partially masked by the pool; **3,** profile: obvious; **a,** polyp dome image; **b,** stalk implantation into the dome; **c,** stalk implantation into the wall

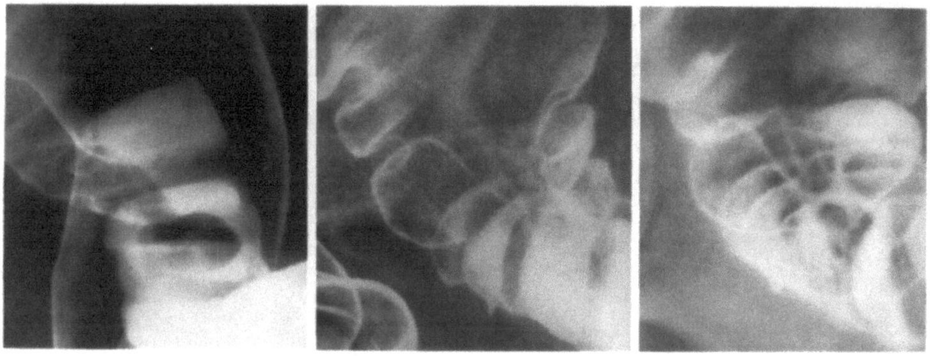

A, B, C

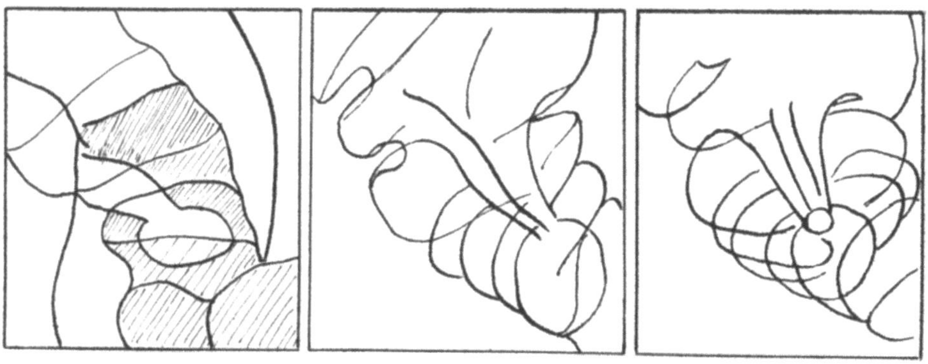

A, B, C

Fig. 3.21. Pedunculated polyp: **A,** filling defect; **B, C,** here it is the stalk which is especially visible; it crosses the transversal lines of the haustra

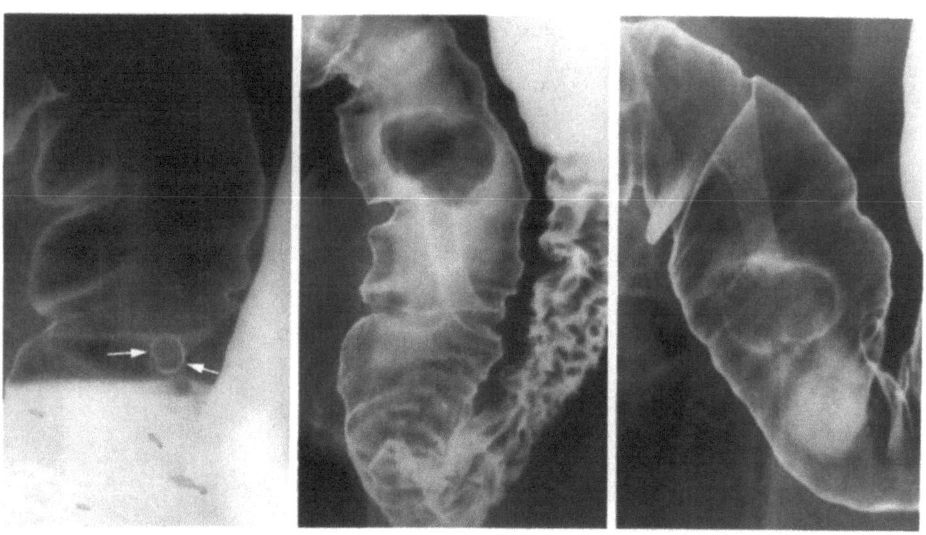

A, B, C

Fig. 3.22. Long-stalked polyp: **A,** only the stalk is seen *(arrow)*. The rest of the polyp is masked by barium; **B,** filling defect; **C,** another double contrast view shows a change in position. The long stalk makes for high mobility

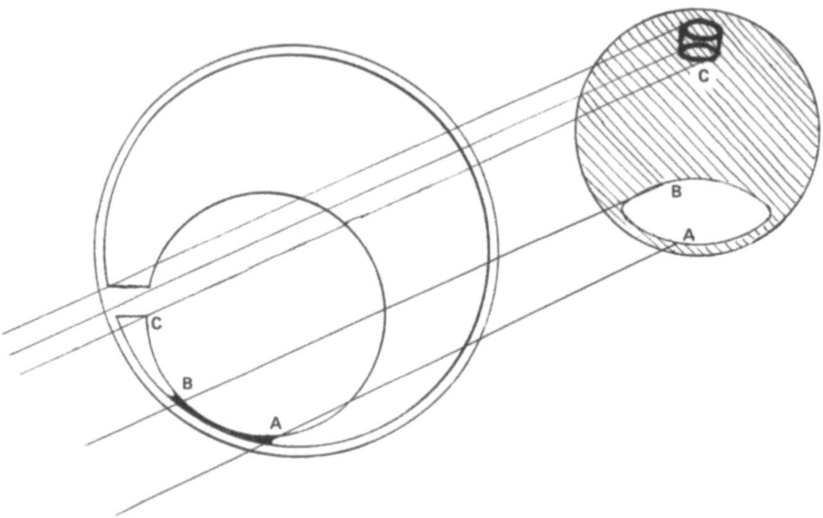

Fig. 3.23. Diagrammatic representation of a double-base image. **A, B,** the area of contact between the dome and wall may be mistaken for the base. **C,** polyp base

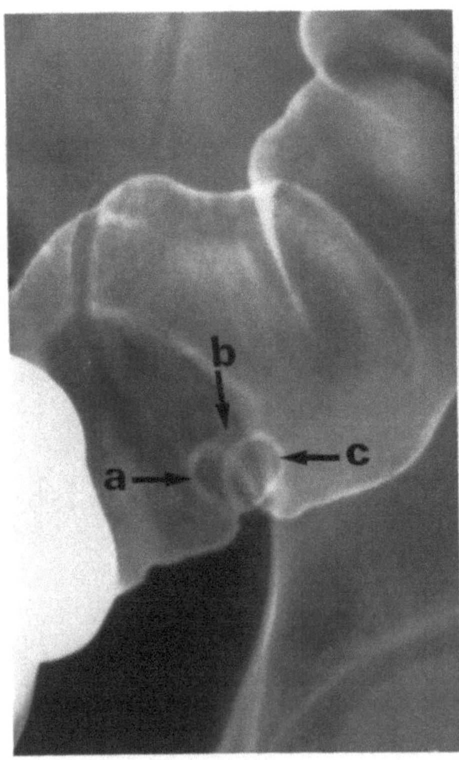

3.24

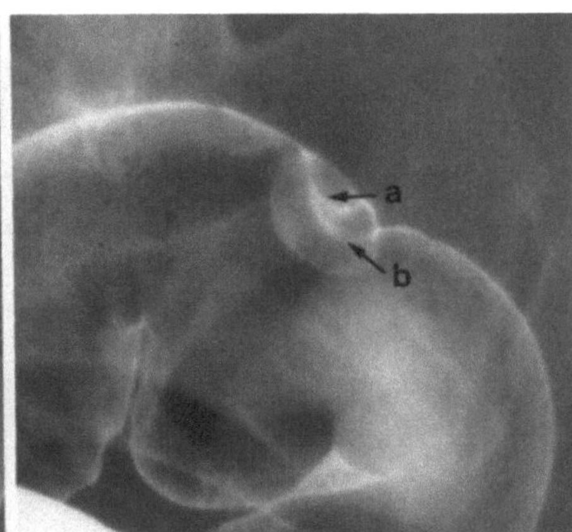

3.25

Fig. 3.24. Example of a double-base image for a sessile polyp: **a,** polyp base; **b,** polyp dome; **c,** circle of contact

Fig. 3.25. Intermediate polyp, double-base image: **a,** true base; **b,** contact between polyp and wall

3.2.3 Diagnostic Problems

3.2.3.1 Differential Diagnosis of Polyps

Perfect bowel preparation is necessary to show the images described above.

Severe fecal stasis (Fig. 3.26) is represented by multiple filling defects or a "blotchy" appearance. It should be detected in the plain abdominal radiograph or, at worst, at the beginning of the filling phase when confronted with free filling defects "carried by the barium stream." It is useless to continue the examination.

Moderate fecal stasis cannot always be detected before the examination. It is represented either by semiliquid adherent matter coating the walls (cf. Chap. 2) or often as free multiple ring shadows (Fig. 3.27) as seen in films performed in

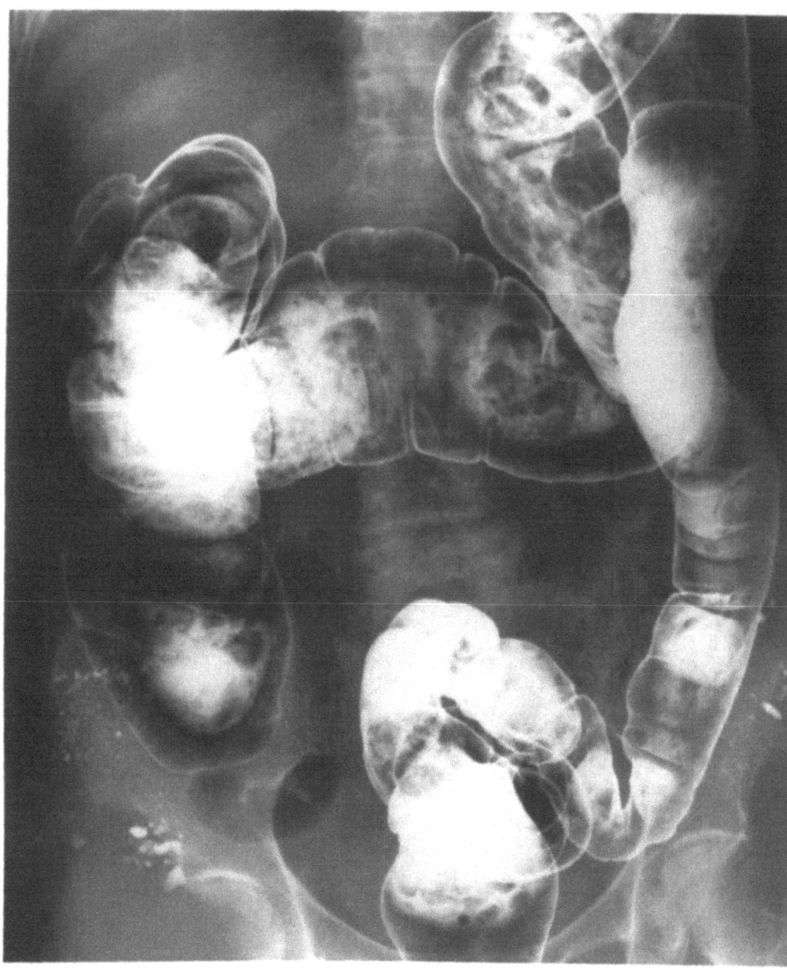

Fig. 3.26. Severe fecal stasis. With the patient in the supine position, numerous filling defects, most visible in barium pools, make interpretation impossible

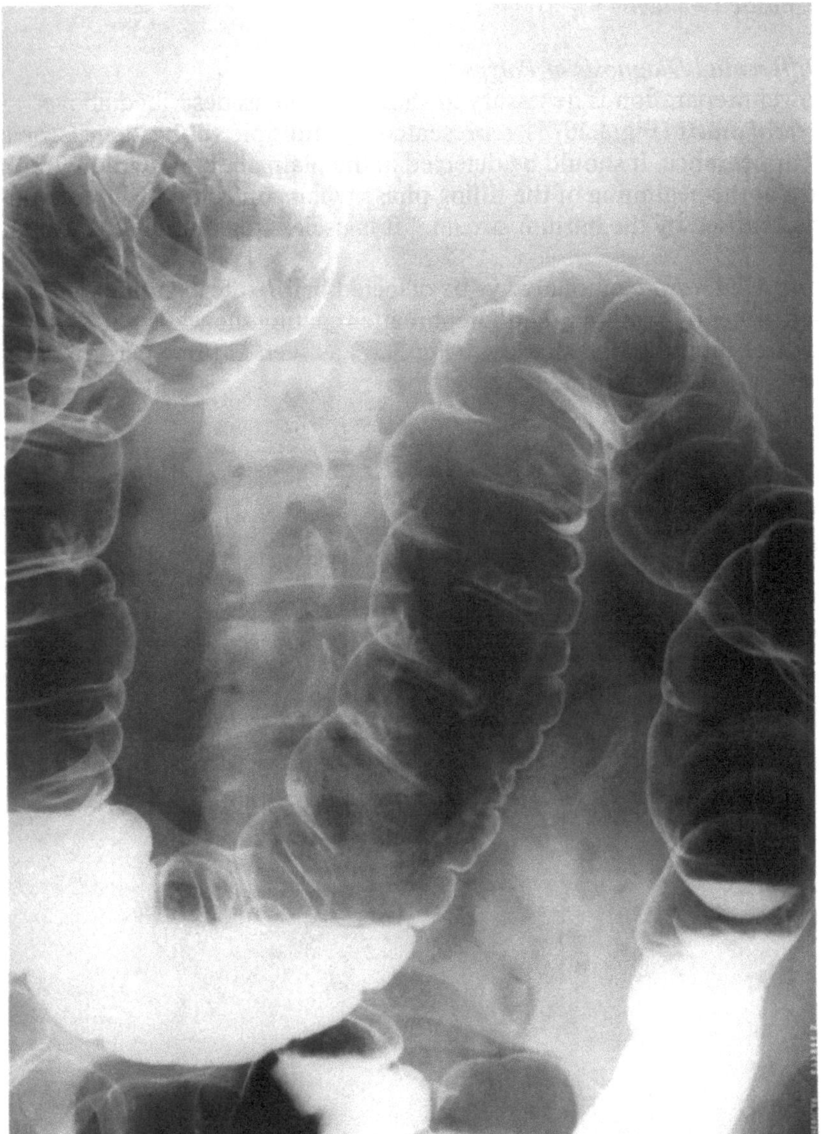

Fig. 3.27. Another patient. In the upright position, many ring shadows persist. Despite their angled and blurred contours, their number makes interpretation impossible

the upright position. (The examination can sometimes be interpreted as the fecal residue descends in the barium.) Fecal residue is seen as filling defects in the pool. The examination cannot be interpreted if there is much fecal residue. In practice, when the examination is performed well, the ring shadow most often attracts attention and alerts the examiner to check for the lesion in other radiographs.

A ring shadow may represent a polyp, fecal matter, bubbles, or an obstructed diverticulum.

Adherent fecal matter is often irregular in form, with angled contours surrounded by a dense, blurred line (Fig. 3.28). The best way to distinguish between fecal matter and polyps is to show the polyp dome from a three-quarter view or in profile. If this is unsuccessful and if the image is seen in several radiographs, its exact nature is doubtful, requiring either a second double contrast enema or an endoscopic examination.

Air bubbles are rare and are often joined together in more or less free clusters (Fig. 3.29). Oil droplets are perfectly spherical and equally mobile (Fig. 3.30).

Obstructed diverticula may form circular images with relatively clear centers. The radiograph taken in profile is fundamental since it may show, the image at the top of a haustration, a fine barium line penetrating the diverticulum and visible outside the colonic lumen, or absence of the "hat sign" (see Chap. 8). There may, however, still be some doubt at the end of the examination.

The target image and even hat sign may occur for a diverticulum seen frontally or from a three-quarter view, depending on whether it has a large or narrow neck. In order to differentiate it from an intermediate polyp or stalk, the following are checked: sharpness of the base circle (often blurred or associated with a double-base image for polyps); radiologic density, which is often greater for diverticula (since they retain barium); whether the diverticulum eventually fills; the presence of a fluid level in the upright position; any change in form during the examination; the radiograph taken in profile which places the lesion outside the lumen; orientation of the top of the image toward the periphery of the colonic segment; and absence of a filling defect in the pool.

It becomes particularly difficult when diverticula are numerous since it is difficult to find them on additional radiographs with different incidences. It is certainly true in cases of diverticulosis that most polyps go undetected with double contrast. Changes in haustral folding add to the problems of interpretation.

The image of a sessile polyp seen in profile may be simulated by two opaque artifacts: the barium droplet and the mucus on the colonic wall. (The twisted and stringy form of mucus and its characteristic density make it easily recognizable.)

The image of a polyp with a long stalk may also be simulated by a mucus strand suspended from the wall (see Chap. 2).

The image of a polyp seen frontally may, in certain cases, be simulated by a vein stone (phlebolith) superimposed on the colon (Fig. 3.31).

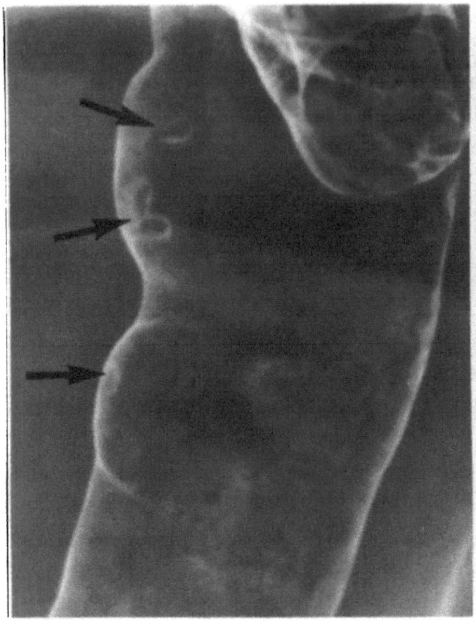

3.28

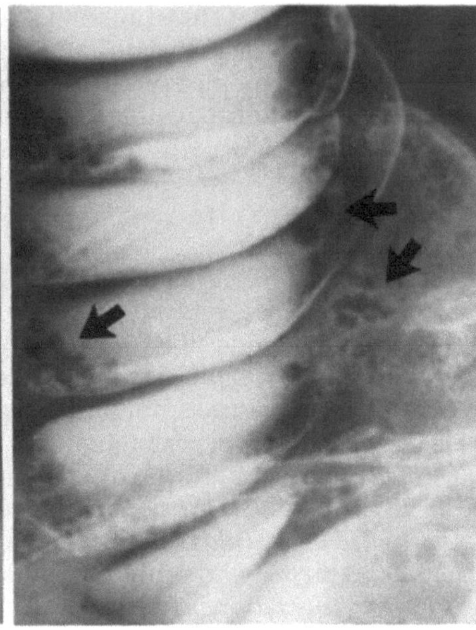

3.29

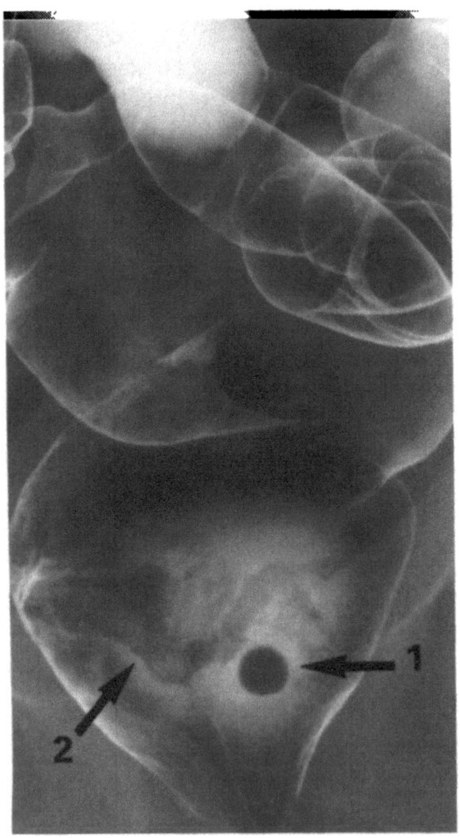

3.30

Fig. 3.28. Adherent fecal matter *(arrows)* usually: (1) has uneven, angular contours; (2) is surrounded by a blurred line; (3) is heterogeneous; and (4) is without the hat sign

Fig. 3.29. Air bubbles *(arrows)* are spherical, joined together, and mobile (they are rare with Rhodorsil)

Fig. 3.30. Spherical oil droplets *(arrow 1)* are mobile (castor oil orally should not be used and the nozzle should be lubricated with a water soluble lubricant). Note the nearby "mucus bundle" *(arrow 2)*. These two images will vary in later radiographs

Fig. 3.31. Calcification simulating a polyp. **A,** here the image is rounded and dense, and is projected on the intermarginal aspect of the rectum; **B,** in a strict frontal radiograph the opacity is projected outside the rectum; in this case it is a vein stone

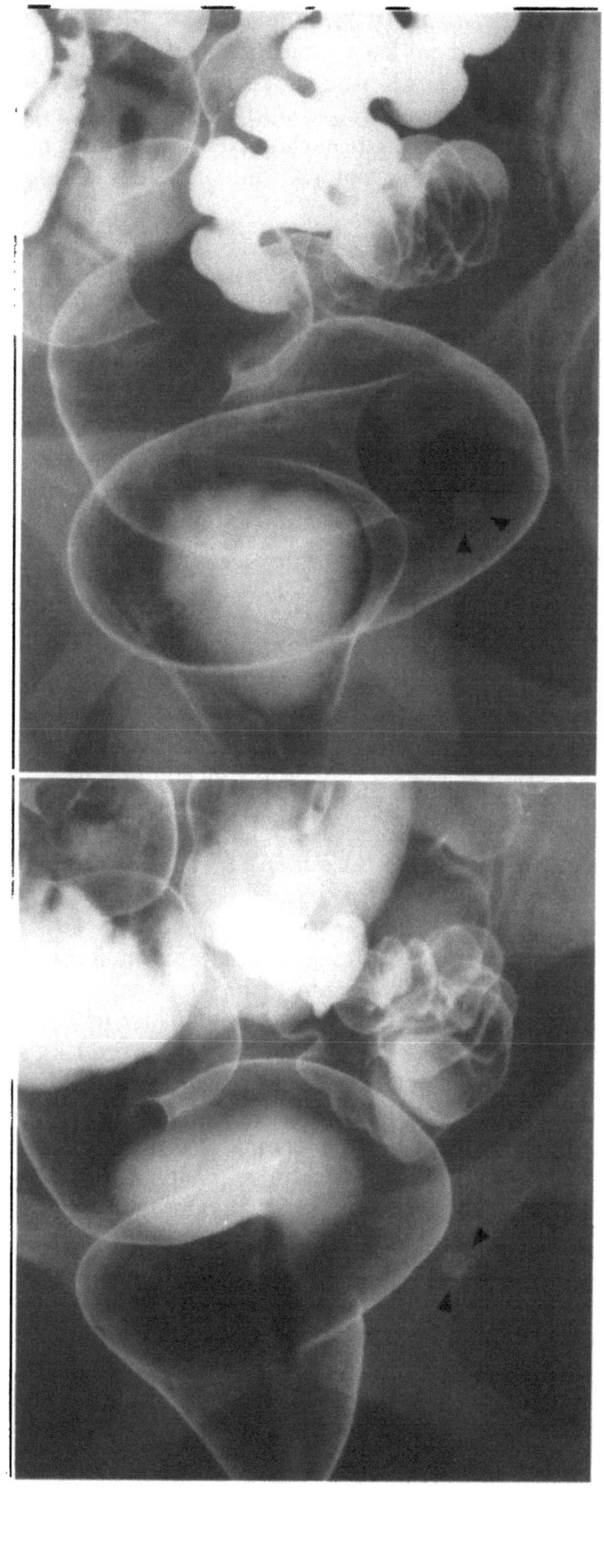

A

B

3.2.3.2 Reliability of Polyp Images

In practice, the different basic images described above (hat sign; filling defect; ring shadow, target, and stalk images) are not equally reliable in the diagnosis of polyps. A retrospective study of the analysis of 200 polyp images verified by endoscopic examination showed an important nuance in formulating the radiologic diagnosis of polyps. This diagnosis should be formulated as positive or only probable [15].

3.2.3.3 Positive Diagnosis

We may be certain when confronted with signs whose predictive value in diagnosing polyps approaches 1. They include any of the basic images whose size is greater than 1 cm (provided the colon is correctly prepared); a stalk image; a ring shadow or filling defect with polycyclic contours; a target image when a diverticulum can be ruled out; and the association of three basic images (for example, filling defect + circle image + hat sign) in the different radiographs. A diagnosis of polyps is certain when any of these signs are present. Thus, in the case of a negative endoscopic examination, a new short-term radiologic examination is necessary.

3.2.3.4 Uncertain Diagnosis

In other cases a diagnosis of polyps can only be made with a certain probability. Here, endoscopic examination is called for and will be more easily accepted if negative. Again, the predictive value of the basic images in diagnosing polyps must be considered separately: hat sign 0.81; filling defect with sharp borders, 0.76; profile image, 0.60; and ring shadow with sharp borders, 0.55. The art of the radiologist is to transform a probable diagnosis into a positive one, if this is the case, by changing the angle of incidence during the examination as soon as a suggestive image is seen and by carefully studying the resulting radiographs.

3.2.3.5 Recognizing Artifacts

Our study has also made it possible to make a better diagnosis of artifacts, of which three images seem to be characteristic: the piriform image (grape pit form), which has a predictive value close to 1 for diagnosing artifacts; angular contour image (Fig. 3.28), 0.90; and blurred ring shadow, 0.92. While results of this study are incomplete, they have made it possible to improve the method's reliability by reducing the number of false positives. Since the goal of the double contrast barium enema is the detection of polyps, an effort must be made to reduce excessive false positives, requiring unnecessary, time-consuming, and expensive endoscopic examinations. Thus, it is the responsibility of all radiologists to verify the values we propose by checking the degree of false negative endoscopic examinations with endoscopists. The radiologist can make his own rough evaluation according to the frequency of polyps in the population and in radiologic reports.

3.3 Colonic Polyposis

Colonic polyposis poses several problems for the radiologist. The first is nosologic: confronted with a number of polyps, at what point do we begin talking about polyposis? The second is diagnostic: how do we recognize polyposis and differentiate it from other similar diseases?

Definition of Polyposis. The frequent multiplicity of polyps (one out of four cases; Fig. 3.32) makes the problem difficult. For some authors [2–10], discovery of more than two polyps and a marked tendency for recurrence suggest a diagnosis of polyposis. For others more than 100 polyps are necessary. We re-

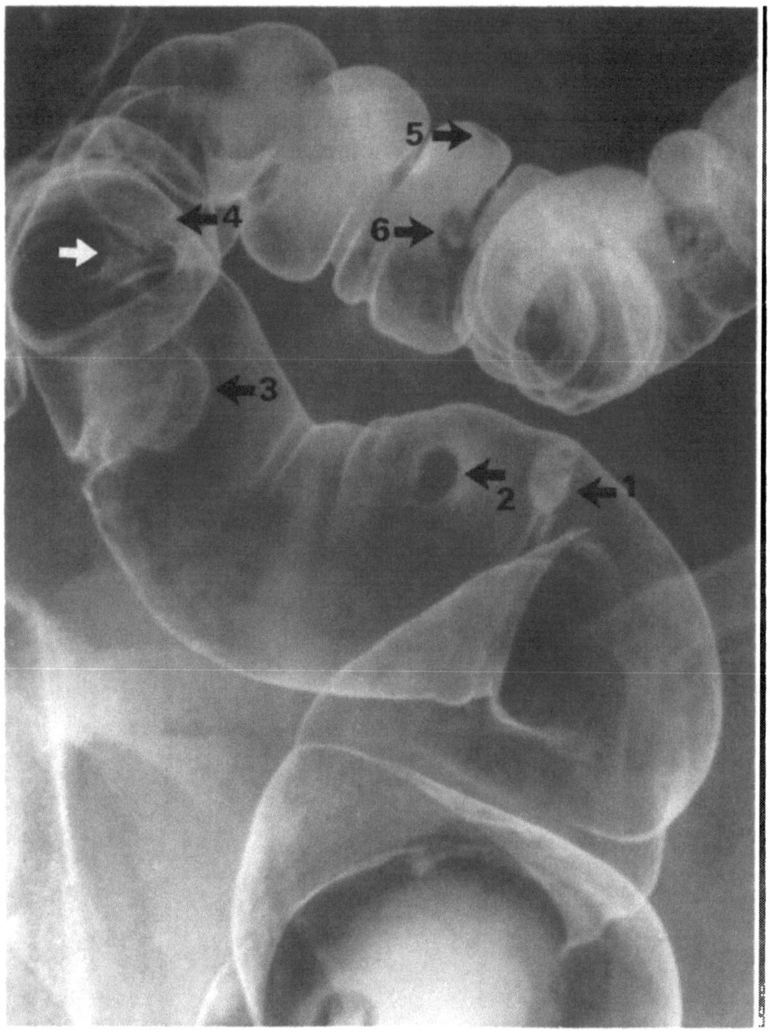

Fig. 3.32. Multiple polyps (25% of polyps are multiple). In this radiograph, four polyps (**1, 2, 3, 4**) were visible; two went unnoticed (**5, 6**)

serve the term polyposis for patients having innumerable polyps and use the term multiple polyps for those which can still be counted. This purely macroscopic definition involves neither the histologic nature nor the possible familial character of the disease, both of which are essential elements for any therapeutic decision.

Diagnostic Aspects of Polyposis. Two diagnostic aspects can be described according to the stage of development: the appearance of early-stage polyposis and that of advanced polyposis.

3.3.1 Early-Stage Polyposis

Early-stage polyposis is represented by very small sessile polyps seen radiologically as clearly ring shadows. They are so flat that they are rarely seen in profile (Fig. 3.33). They may also be represented by round, clearly limited filling defects seen in a pool (Fig. 3.34). These appearances may be found either separately during familial surveys or adjacent to more evolved polyps (Fig. 3.35).

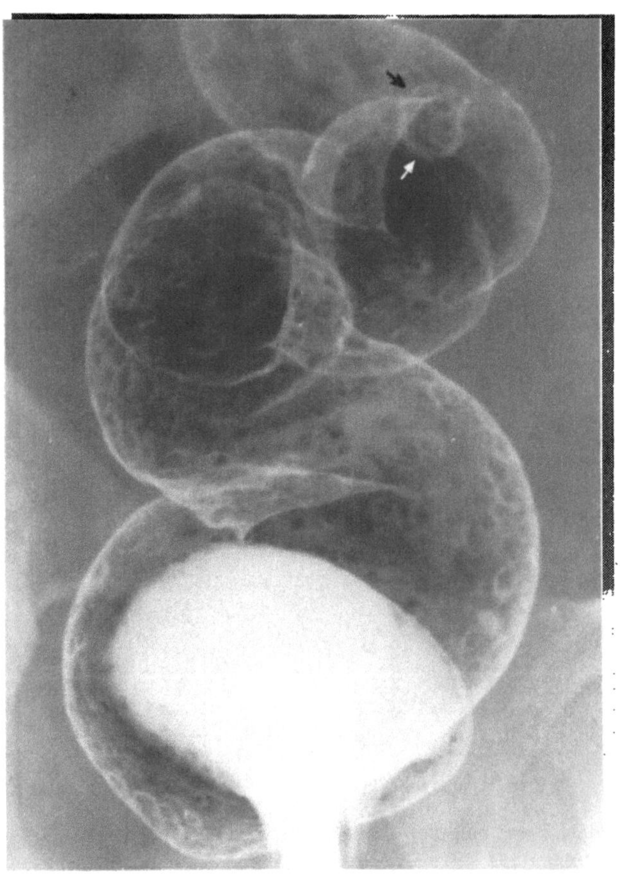

Fig. 3.33. Familial adenomatous polyposis: new lesions on the rectum are associated with a larger intermediate polyp *(arrows).* Note the finely circled character of the images

Differential Diagnosis. There are essentially three possiblities:

1. Adherent fecal matter is small in size with blurred, irregular, and angular contours.

2. Lymphoid nodular hyperplasia (or colorectal lymphoid follicular pattern) can be mistaken for polyposis from the radiographic study, resulting in unnecessary colectomies if preliminary histologic verification is not obtained [3]. The radiologic appearance of lymphoid nodular hyperplasia which is easily recognizable in children since it occurs in one out of three examinations, is less evident in adults. Nodular images 1-3 mm in diameter with blurred borders are seen on the colonic walls in an otherwise normal double contrast study (Fig. 3.36). This appearance is found particularly on radiographs obtained with the patient in the upright position at the end of the examination.

3. Certain cases of colitis in the early or cicatricial stage, whether it be Crohn's disease or pseudomembranous colitis, have a nodular, studded appearance approaching that of lymphoid nodular hyperplasia (Figs. 3.37, 3.38). Here again the blurred character of the images makes it possible to differentiate between these and true polyps. Diagnosis may be much more difficult at the cicatricial stage. Small ring shadows could be mistaken for polyposis unless other telltale signs of polyposis are present: sometimes branched digital polyps, haustral abnormalities, previous history, or ulcerations on a nearby or distant colonic segment (Fig. 3.39). In the absence of these elements, an endoscopic examination is essential.

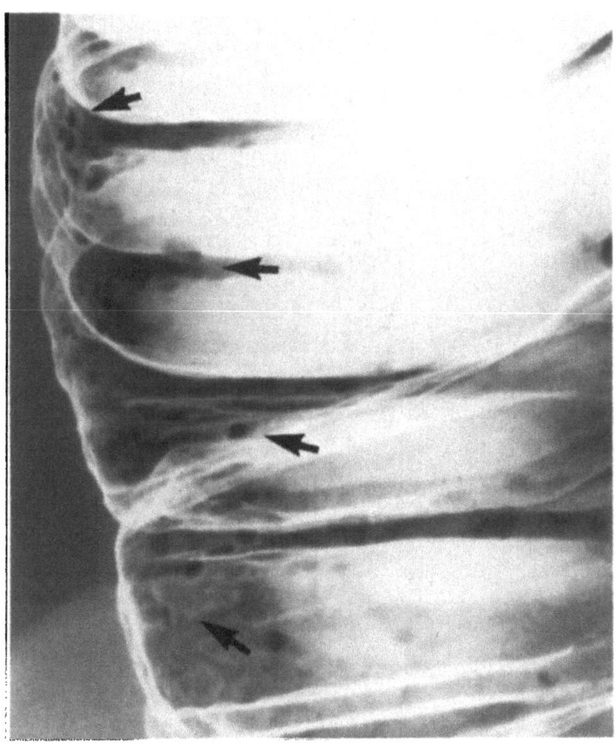

Fig. 3.34. Early-stage adenomatous polyposis in the ascending colon. Note the regular filling defects in the pool. Image size varies and the arrangement of the images is irregular

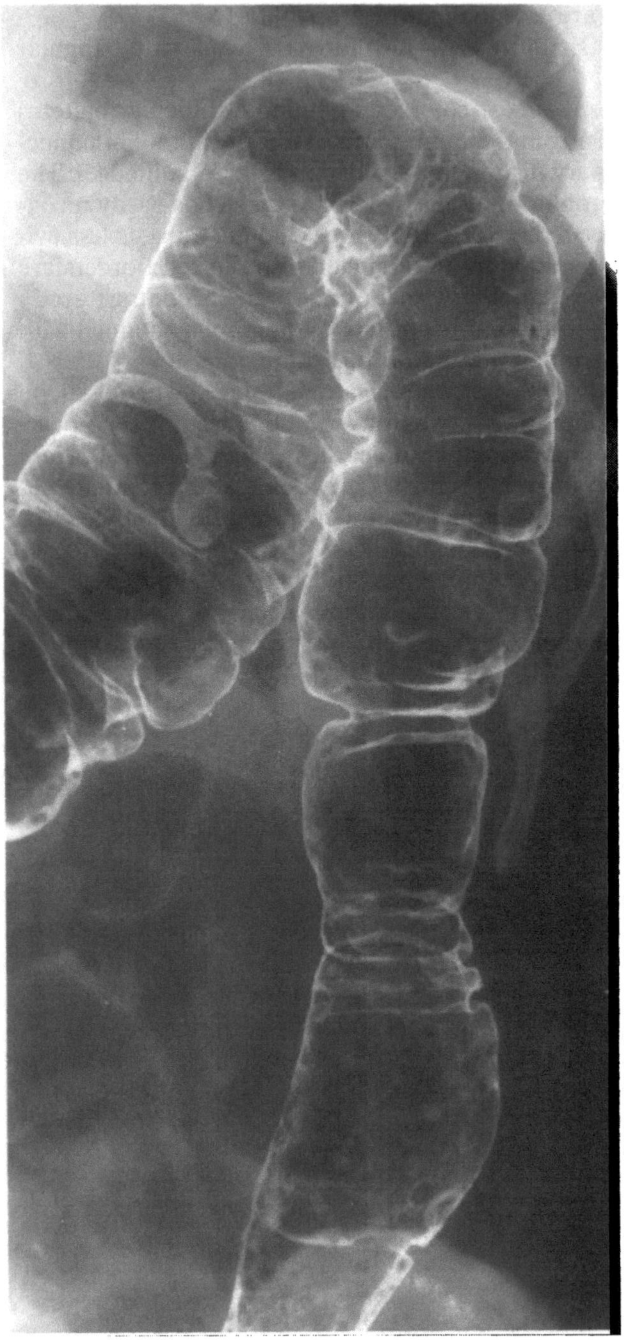

Fig. 3.35. Early-stage adenomatous polyposis: association of early-stage and advanced lesions (pedunculated)

▷
Fig. 3.37. Image simulating early-stage polyposis: clear disseminated images 2-4 mm in diameter, of variable size and contour found in the splenic flexure above ulcerated proctitis. Biopsy: nonspecific interstitial colitis

▷
Fig. 3.38. Image simulating early-stage polyposis. Radiologically: studded appearance of the rectum. Endoscopically: false membranes suggesting early-stage pseudomemranous colitis. Recent use of antibiotic. Histologically: erosive rectocolitis. Complete regression with vancomycin

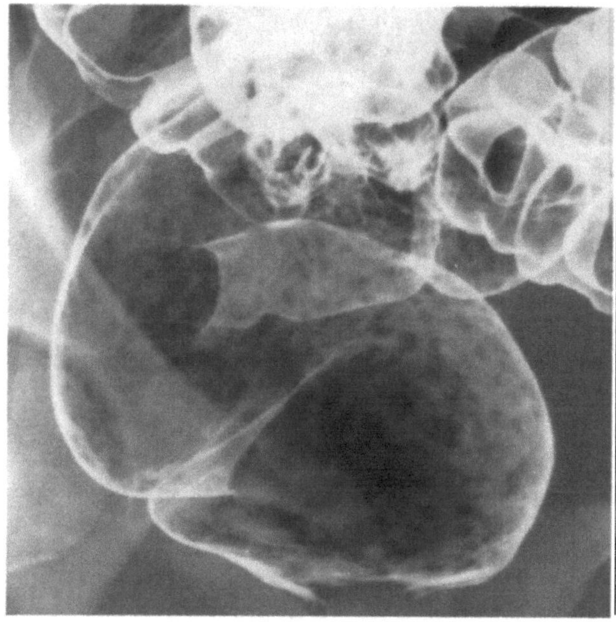

Fig. 3.36. Rectal lymphoid follicular pattern. The small size and blurred border is highly suggestive. Histologic study will confirm it

3.37

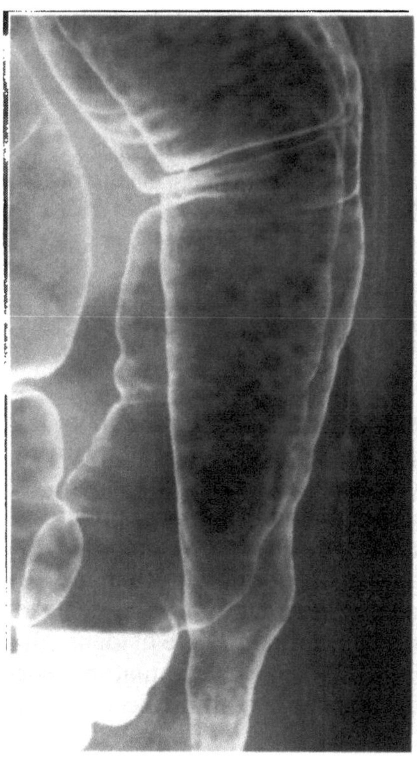

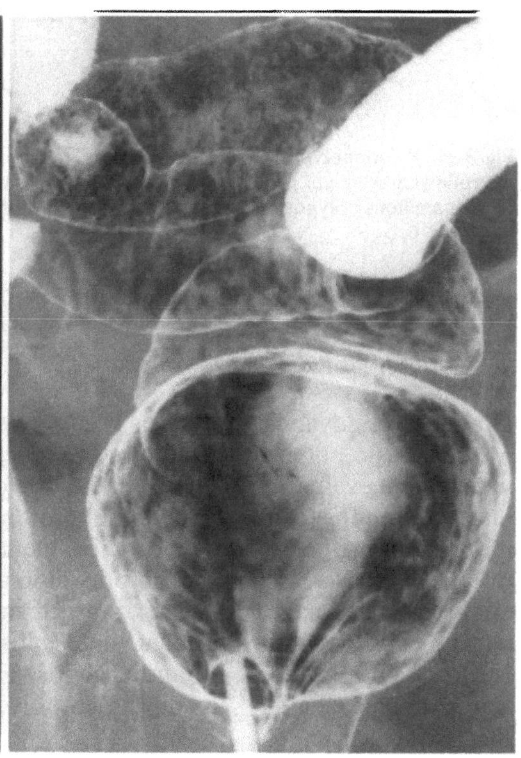

3.38

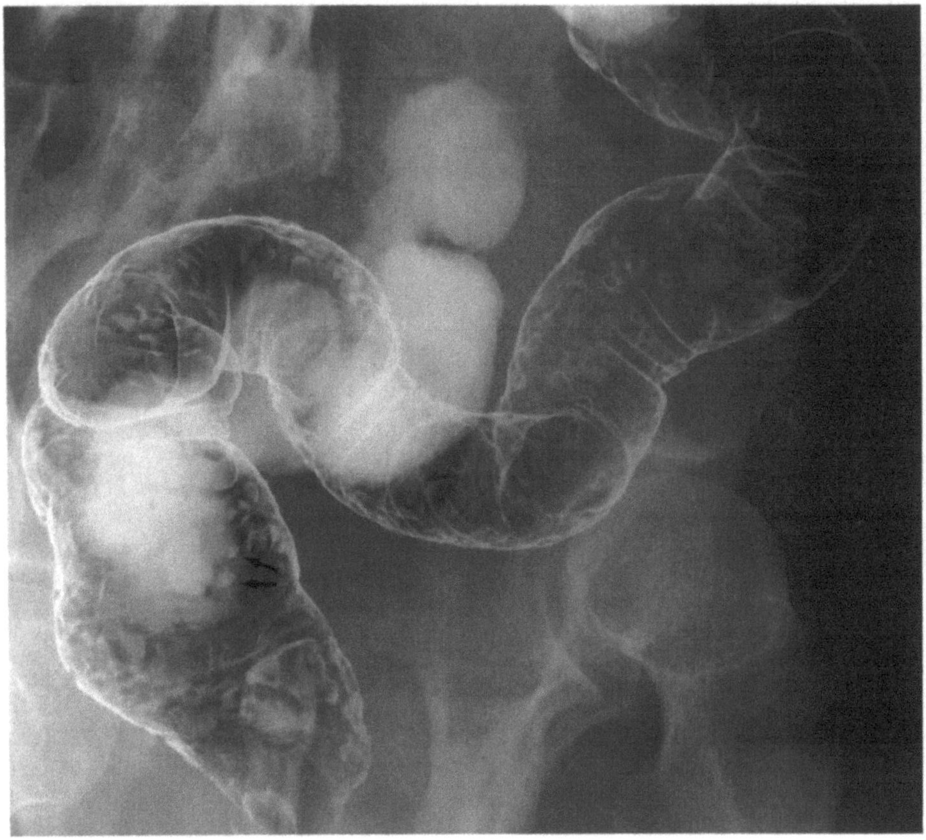

Fig. 3.39. Pseudopolyposis in ulcerative colitis. This appearance might pose a diagnostic problem if the following were not present: (1), ulcerations *(arrows)*; (2), diverse polyp forms, unusual in cases of adenomatous polyposis; (3), previous history (radiology and endoscopy)

3.3.2 Advanced Polyposis

Diagnosis of advanced polyposis is easier when the coexistence of more or less evolved basic polyp images is present (Figs. 3.40, 3.41). Double contrast provides for an evaluation of the spread of the disease (segmentary or generalized) and its adjoining (diffused polyposis) or nonadjoining (disseminated polyposis) nature. Among possible diagnostic problems are: (1) The poorly prepared colon: the diagnosis rests on the mobility of images in the upright position and fine analysis of the images (absence of target, stalk, or indentation images). (2) Advanced colitis is rarely a problem since haustral abnormalities are evident. This is the case of pseudomembranous colitis (Fig. 3.42) or postinflammatory pseudopolyps (see Chap. 4) seen during chronic inflammatory colitis (ulcerative colitis, Crohn's disease ...).

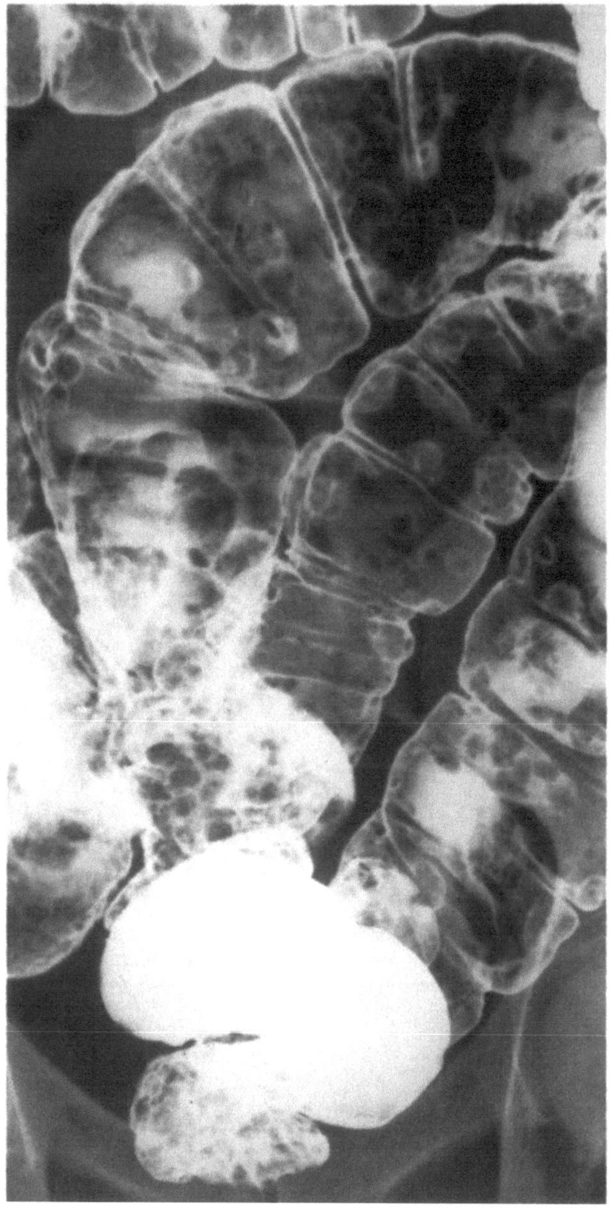

Fig. 3.40. Advanced adenomatous polyposis. This appearance might suggest a "dirty" colon. Fine analysis leaves no doubt

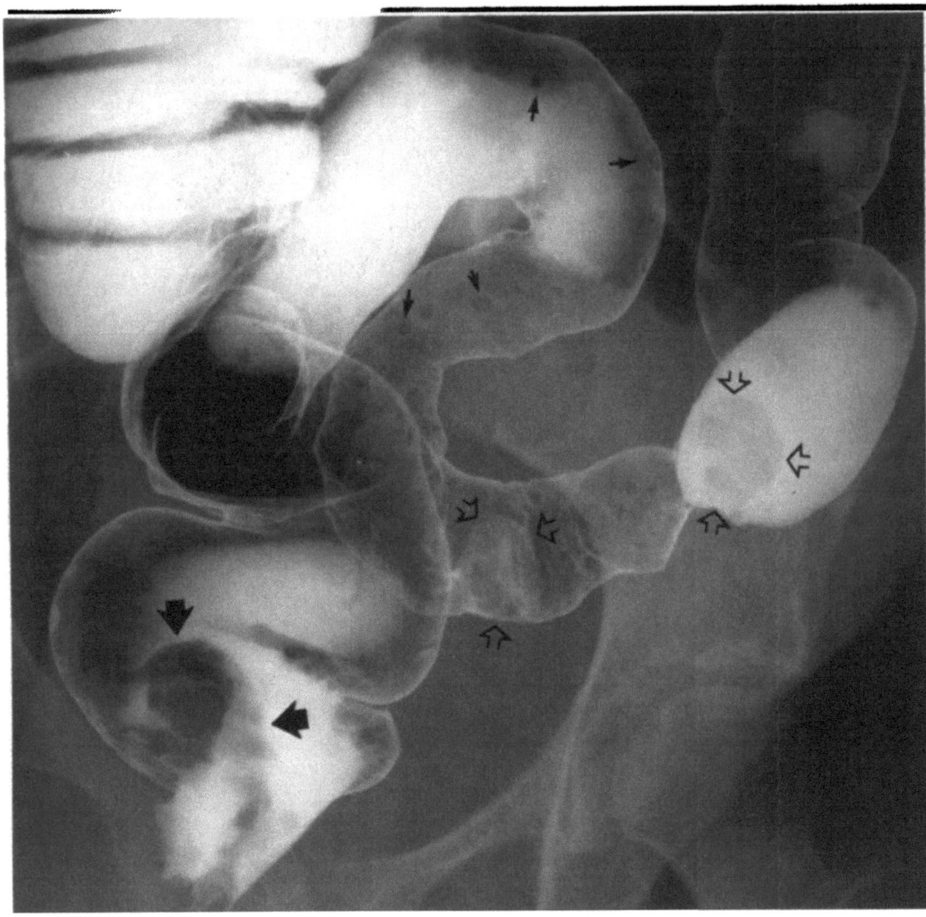

Fig. 3.41. Advanced adenomatous polyposis (malignant change). Note the association of: ulcerated rectal cancer *(large arrows);* multiple sessile micropolyps (several are designated by *small arrows*); two larger already degenerated polyps *(open arrows)*

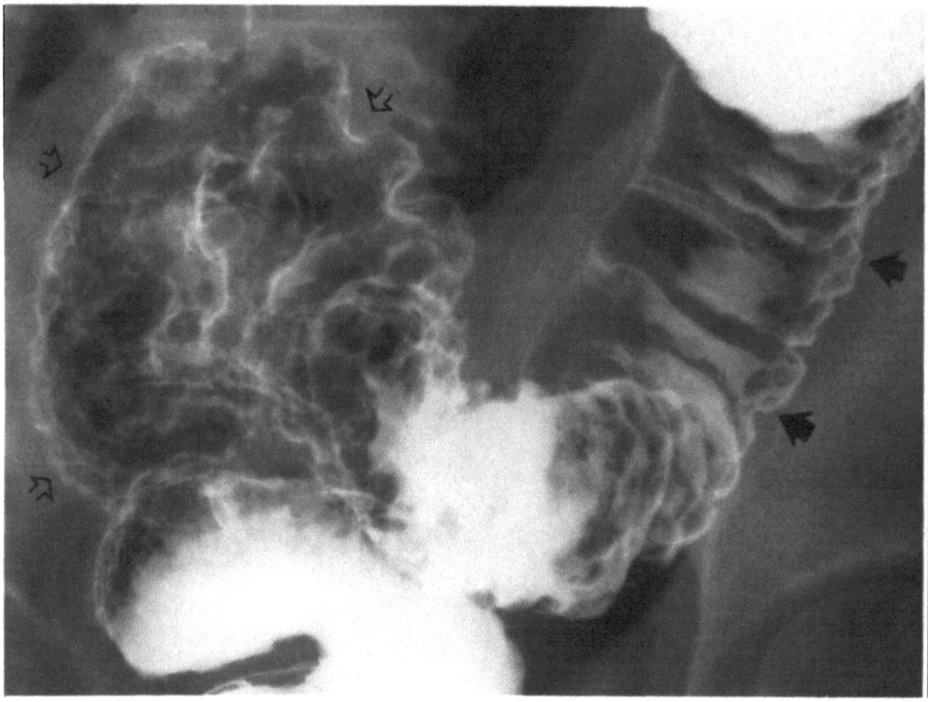

Fig. 3.42. Clindamycine pseudomembranous colitis. Polypoid images *(large arrows)* with caliber, haustral, and mucosal abnormalities *(open arrows)* (Courtesy of Dr. Regent, Nancy)

3.3.3 Appearances Specific to Certain Polyposis Syndromes

Certain polyposis syndromes may have specific appearances in view of their histologic nature: (1) Adenomatous polyposis, when discovered in the stage of malignant change (Fig. 3.41), appears as advanced cancer. (2) In intestinal cystic pneumatosis, intraparietal air bubbles are found in contact with polypoid images; these fit perfectly on the polypoid images (like the pieces of a puzzle) and may be associated with a polyhedral appearance of the colonic contours (Figs. 3.43, 3.44). The radiologic diagnosis can thus be positively affirmed [12]. (3) More difficult is the diagnosis of malignant lymphomatous polyps. These are suspected when the radiologist is confronted with the submucous appearance of polyps which look more like polypoid swellings of the folds (Fig. 3.45). This image, however, is not found in all cases of lymphomatous polyps.

In conclusion, a general rule should be remembered: double contrast will suffice for a positive diagnosis and will diagnose the spread of polyposis but not its histologic nature. This is for the pathologist to confirm.

No therapeutic decision can be made without the preliminary histologic examination of one or several polyps.

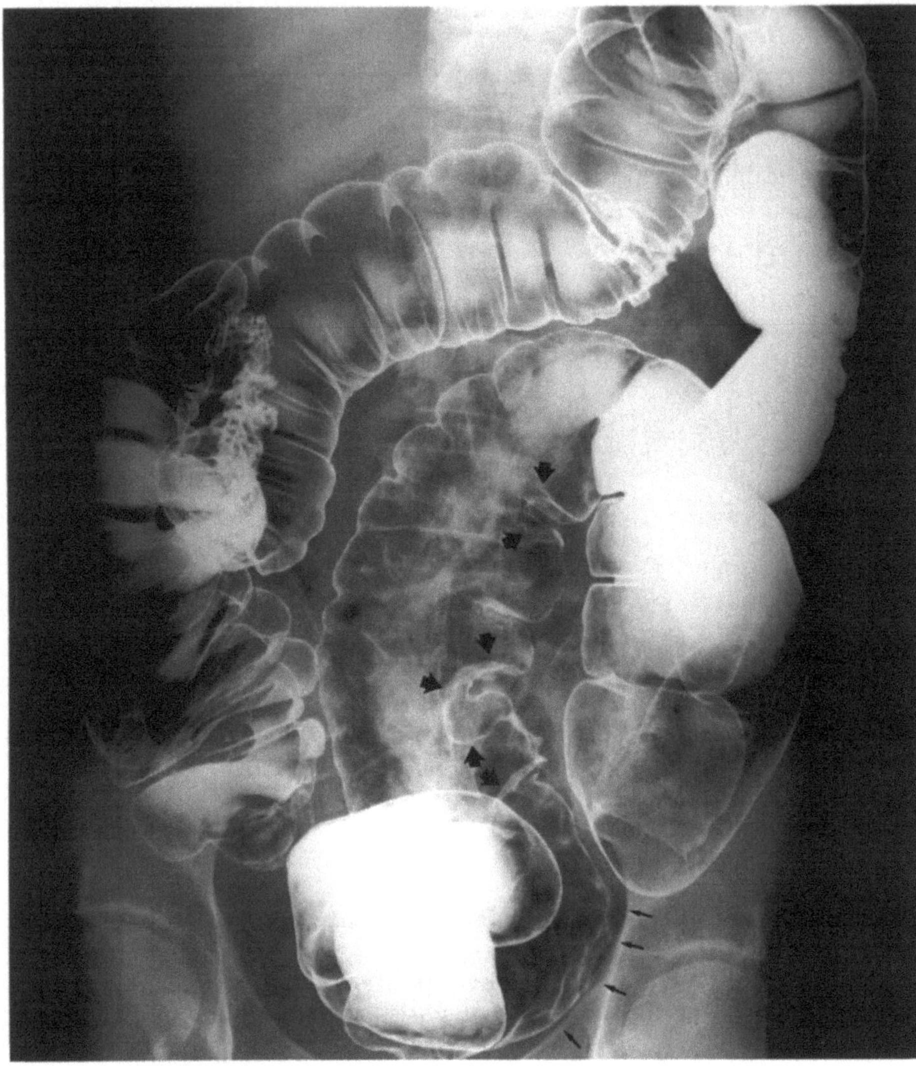

Fig. 3.43. Cystic pneumatosis in the sigmoid: polypoid images of variable form and submucous appearance (gradually joining the wall) *(arrows)*

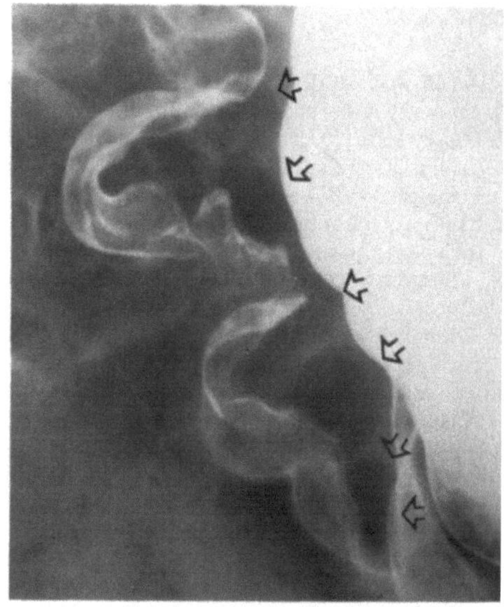

Fig. 3.44. Intraparietal gaseous images (extraluminal: *open arrows*) on polypoid images which affirm the diagnosis of cystic pneumatosis

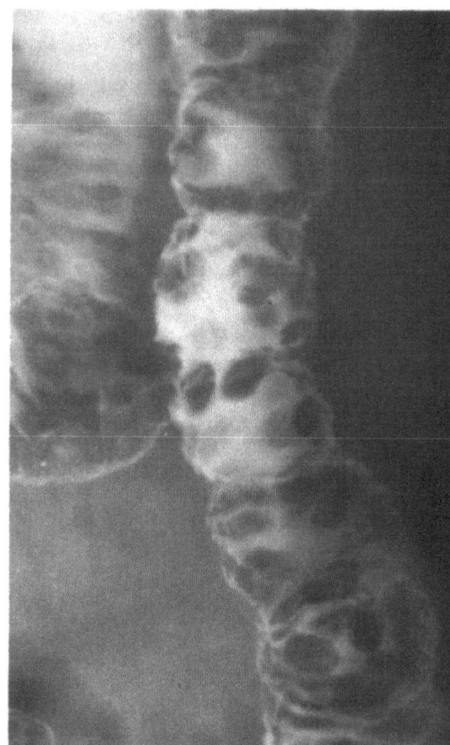

Fig. 3.45. Malignant lymphomatous polyposis: in the descending colon polyps appear as regular filling defects and in the transverse colon as polypoid defects of haustral folds. (Courtesy of Dr. Chavanne, Paris)

References

1. Ament AE, Alfidi RJ, Rad PS (1982) Basal indentation of sessile polypoid lesions. A function of geometry rather than a sign of malignancy. Radiology 143: 341-344
2. Bussey HJR (1975) Familial polyposis. John Hopkins - London
3. Collins JO, Falk M, Guibone R (1966) Benign lymphoid polyposis of the colon: a case report. Pediatric 38: 897-899
4. Ekelund G, Lindstrom C, Rosengren JE (1974) Appearance and growth of early carcinomas of the colon and rectum. Acta Radiol 15: 670-679
5. Gilbersten VA (1974) Proctosigmoidoscopy and polypectomy in reducing the incidence of rectal cancer. Cancer (Suppl) 34: 936-939
6. Grinnell RS (1964) The chance of cancer and lymphatic metastasis in small colon tumors discovered on X ray examination. Ann Surg 159: 132-138
7. Laufer I, Smith NC, Mullens JE (1976) The radiological demonstration of colorectal polyps undetected by endoscopy. Gastroenterology 70: 167-170
8. Marti R, Descombes J (1976) Intérêt de la radiographie en double contraste dans le dépistage des polypes recto-coliques. Arch Fr Mal App Dig 65: 197-200
9. Miller RE, Skucas J (1983) The radiological examination of the colon. Nijhoff, Amsterdam pp 217-242
10. Morson B (1974) The polyp cancer sequence of the large bowel. Proc Roy Soc Med 67: 451-457
11. Potet F, Soulard J (1973) Anatomo-pathologie et modalités évolutives spontanées des polypes et polyposes coliques. Rev Prat 23: 2219-2235
12. Riche MC, Weissman A, Menault JY, Elbim A, Grellet J (1977) Pneumatose kystique à localisation sigmoïdienne: apports respectifs de la mucographie colique (lavement en double contraste) et de l'endoscopie. A propos de un cas. J Radiol Electrol 55: 833-837
13. Soullard J (1975) Proctologie, Masson, Paris
14. Spratt JS, Ackerman LV (1960) Relationship of the size of colonic tumors to their cellular composition and biological behavior. Surg Forum 10: 56
15. Weissman A, Clot M, Grellet J (1977) Règles d'interprétation de la radiologie colique en double contraste Diagnostic des polypes. Gastroentérol Clin Biol 1: 281-296
16. Weissman A, Barge HJ, Clot M, Saigot T, Harriague D, Curet P, Grellet J (1981) Aspect nodulaire lymphoïde rectocolique chez l'adulte. J Radiol 62: 449-455
17. Welin S (1958) Modern trends in diagnostic roentgenology of the colon. Br J Radiol 31: 453-464
18. Welin S, Youker J, Spratt JS (1963) The rates and patterns of growth of 375 tumors of the large intestine and rectum observed serially by double contrast enema study. Am J Roentgenol 90: 673
19. Williams CB, Hunt RM, et al. (1974) Colonoscopy in the management of colon polyps. Birt J Surg 61: 673-682
20. Youkers JE, Welin S (1965) Differentiation of true polypoid tumors of the colon from extraneous material. A new roentgen sign. Radiology 84: 610-615
21. Youkers JE, Welin S, Main B (1968) Computer analysis in the differentiation of benign and malignant lesions of the colon. Radiology 90: 794-797

4 Primary Colorectal Cancer

The traditionally described characteristic appearances of colorectal carcinoma (ulceration and neoplasic stenosis) actually correspond to advanced lesions. In 1962, Potet et al. [8] had the insight to suggest a hypothetical relationship between malignant adenomas and ulcerative carcinoma. This hypothesis is now accepted by most authors [3, 7]. Macroscopically, the change from malignant polyp to vegetative infiltrating and ulcerative carcinoma is perfectly conceivable and can be explained by the necrosis frequently associated with malignant tumors (Fig. 4.1). This evolution has been confirmed numerous times by studies of polyps which have developed into common carcinoma [2–9]. Consequently, the study of radiologic appearances of colorectal cancer has three parts: (1) nonspecific radiologic images of sessile or pedunculated lesions where only a histologic study will diagnose their benign or malignant nature: (2) radiologic signs indicating the malignant nature of a polyp; and (3) the radiologic appearance of more advanced cancers.

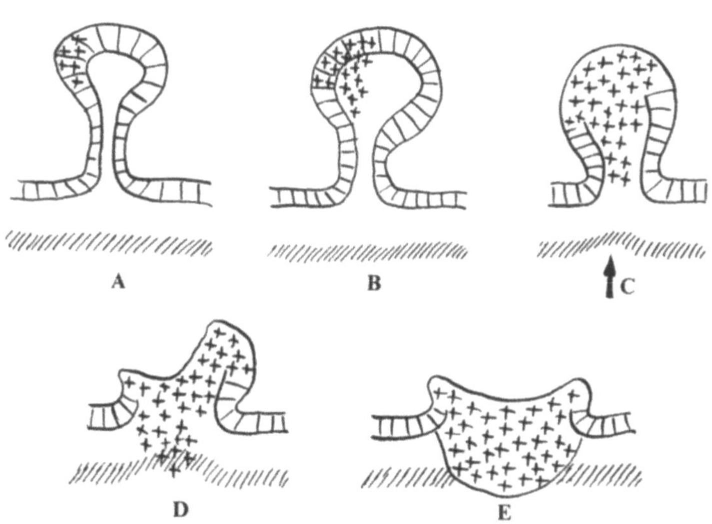

Fig. 4.1. Change from malignant polyp to carcinoma: **A,** intramucosal site of malignant change; **B,** change reaches the polyp axis and penetrates the muscularis mucosae; **C,** change reaches the stalk, which enlarges and shortens; **D,** the malignant change deepens with partial necrosis of the tumor; **E,** "common" malignant ulceration. (Potet [8]). + + + cancer

4.1 Nonspecific Radiologic Appearances of Colorectal Carcinoma

Colorectal carcinoma may have one of the appearances we have described for colorectal polyps: (1) sessile polyp; (2) intermediate polyp; or (3) pedunculated polyp. It may also be found in a carpet-like or polypoid villoma where nothing on the radiographs suggests malignancy. For all these forms, only a histologic study will confirm the malignant nature and spread of the tumor.

4.2 Radiologic Signs Indicating the Malignant Nature of a Polyp

If there is no strict radiologic sign that a lesion is benign, certain images may suggest its malignancy. These signs which must be systematically analyzed are: the size and shape the polyp; an indentation in the base; and possibly the lesion's volume doubling time.

4.2.1 Size

The larger the lesion, the greater its malignant potential. If we use invasive carcinoma as an example (those which have crossed the muscularis mucosae), only 1% of polyps under 1 cm are malignant, 10% between 1 and 2 cm, and 50% over 2 cm [7].

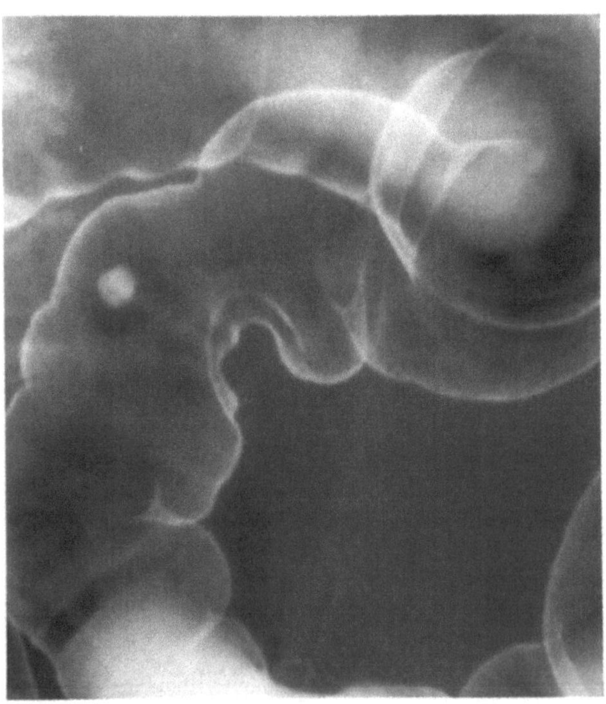

Fig. 4.2. Sessile polypoid lesion with distinct indentation of the base (small carcinoma which infiltrates the wall to the serous membrane)

4.2.2 ***Basal Indentation*** (Fig. 4.2)

According to Welin [12], basal indentation is almost always a sign of malignancy. They noted this in 49% of malignant lesions but also in 4% of benign lesions. This sign, then, is neither specific nor always found for malignant tumors. We believe the development of an indentation is not related to the tumor's parietal spread but more likely to the degree of its circumferential spread.

This hypothesis is shared by others and was even mathematically expressed by Ament [1]. It is frequently the case for villomas in the absence of any malignant change (see Fig. 3.9). For Welin, this indentation is an indication for surgery. In our opinion, a certain distinction should be made. First of all "false" indentations caused by traction of the pedunculated polyp on the wall or stalk (Figs. 4.3, 4.4) and contact between the polyp dome and wall (Figs. 4.5, 4.6) should be differentiated (as described by Welin [12]).

It is only later that endoscopy will determine the different resection possibilities. [Small plateau lesions (Fig. 4.7) may be destroyed by hot biopsy.] For large lesions, however, an indentation is always synonymous with surgery. In these cases, endoscopic resection is impossible.

4.2.3 ***Volume Doubling Time***

No formal conclusion can be made from observing tumor growth in successive studies. It does appear, however, that the faster the growth the greater the chances of malignancy (Welin [12]):

Volume doubling time	percentage of malignant lesions
Greater than 1155 days	1%–2%
1155 to 300 days	19%–29%
Less than 300 days	35%

Growth rates thus estimated are extremely slow and the fastest growing carcinoma took 3 months to increase 2.5 mm in diameter. The rule is to consider any increase in tumor size as an indication for surgery. (This wait-and-see policy is only justifiable for small lesions outside the range of colonoscopy.)

4.2.4 ***Other Signs for Consideration***

The irregular cauliflower appearance of the contours was noted by Welin and Welin [12] in 80% of cancer cases but also in 22% of benign lesions. Cases where the base size is greater than the height are also suspect (Fig. 4.7), but questionable for small lesions [2]. A stalk was noted in 29% of malignant lesions (Fig. 4.4). This is not, then, a strict sign of a benign lesion.

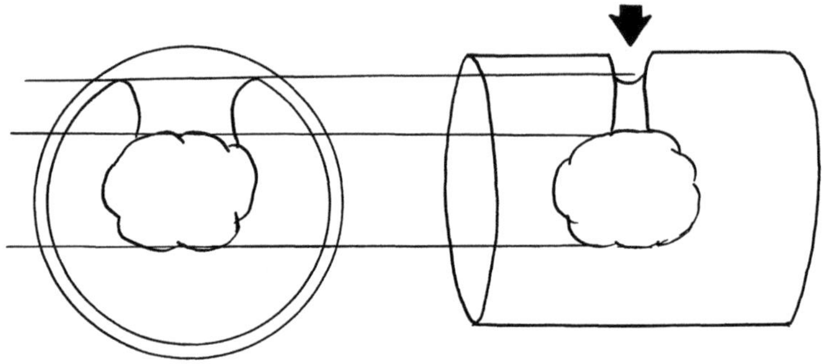

Fig. 4.3. Indentation due to the large size of the stalk and traction of a pedunculated polyp on the wall

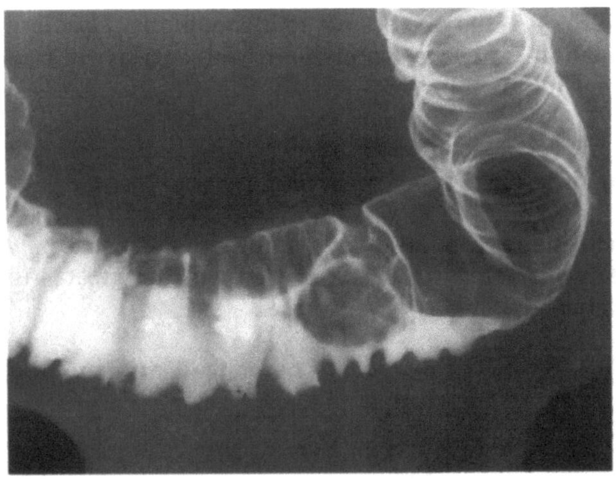

Fig. 4.4. Pedunculated polyp. Indentation here is due only to the large size of the stalk

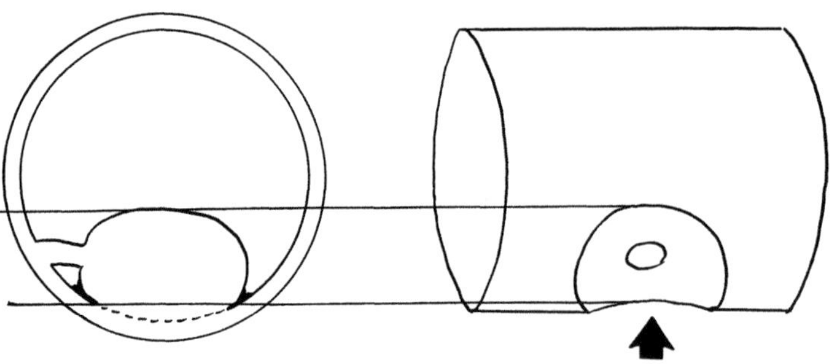

Fig. 4.5. Indentation due to contact between the pedunculated polyp dome and the wall. Barium is driven from the interface dome-wall and accumulates at the periphery around the area of contact. The lesion appears to have a large base, whereas it is really pedunculated

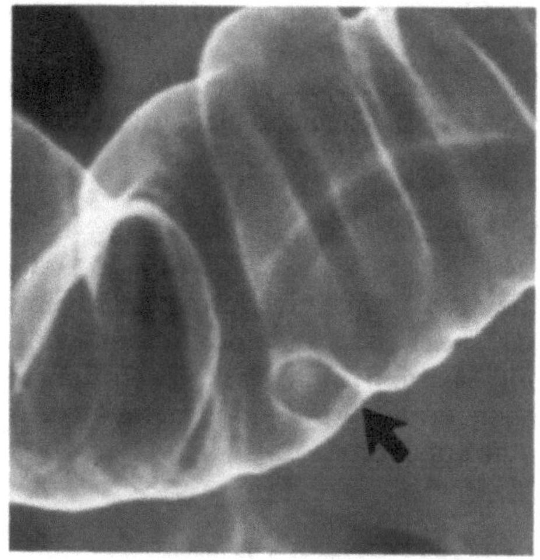

Fig. 4.6. Indentation due to contact between the pedunculated polyp and wall for a small polyp. Endoscopic examination shows it has a short stalk

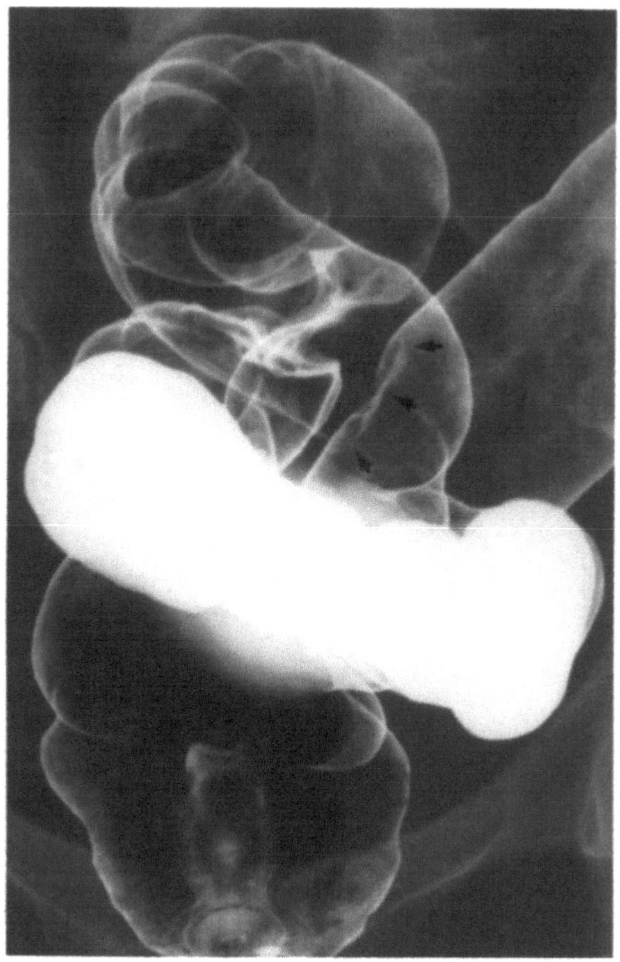

Fig. 4.7. Plateau polyp *(arrows):* this lesion, which is greater in width than height, is suspect. This was a differentiated polyadenoma which could have been removed by hot biopsy

4.3 Classic Appearances of Primary Colorectal Carcinoma

Three classic appearances of advanced carcinoma have been described: (1) vegetative, (2) vegetative ulcerative stenosing or nonstenosing, and (3) infiltrating.

4.3.1 The Strictly Vegetative Form

The strictly vegetative form is relatively rare. Most advanced lesions are ulcerated. These are polypoid lesions with most of the criteria for malignancy (Figs. 4.8, 4.9): large size (greater than 2 cm), irregular contours, and clear basal indentation (certain nondegenerative villomas may, however, have exactly the same appearance.)

4.3.2 The Vegetative Ulcerative and Infiltrating Form

The vegetative ulcerative and infiltrating form is easily the most frequent one. Its radiologic appearance depends essentially on its circumferential spread and degree of bulging into the lumen. The ulceration does not have the same diagnostic importance in double as in single contrast. It is found at the center of a vegetative tumor whose vestiges are at the periphery of the lesion (Fig. 4.10) (peripheral rim of meniscal nonstenosing lesions or tumoral rim of neoplasic stenosis). The vegetative nature of the lesion will be much more evident on the radiographs than its ulcerative nature, which is often shown only after tissue examination. Some have called ulcerated and slightly vegetative forms "plaque-like" or "flat carcinoma." This denomination fails to appreciate the raised na-

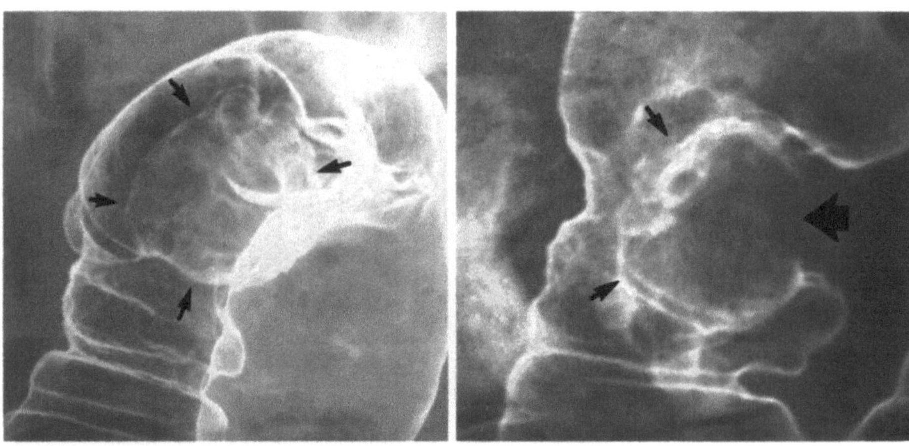

A B

Fig. 4.8. Polypoid form sigmoid adenocarcinoma: **A,** frontally, the lesion which is seen by the tangent und addition effect (see Chap. 2) is projected only in the intermarginal aspect. **B,** in profile the indentation is distinct and the outlines irregular

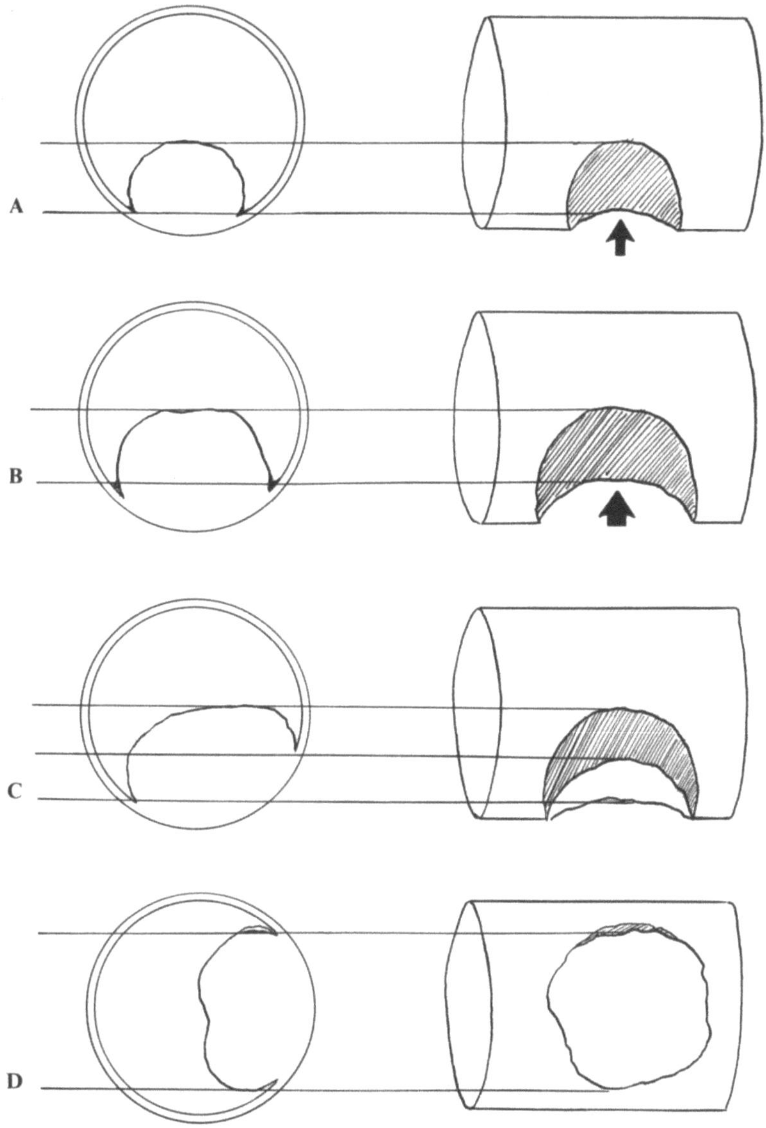

Fig. 4.9. Diagrammatic representation of the radiologic image of vegetative carcinoma according to size and incident angle. **A** Crescent image in strict profile: the internal border of the crescent corresponds to the lesion's dome and the external border to its lateral implantation limits. **B** Increase in the indentation due to an increase in circumferential spread. **C** Quarter of an orange image seen in three-quarter view: the lateral limits of the lesion are no longer superimposed. A quarter of an orange image is thus formed. **D** Frontally if the lesion is not implanted on more than half the circumference, there is no indentation of the colonic margins and the image is projected by the tangent effect in the intermarginal aspect

A

B

C

D

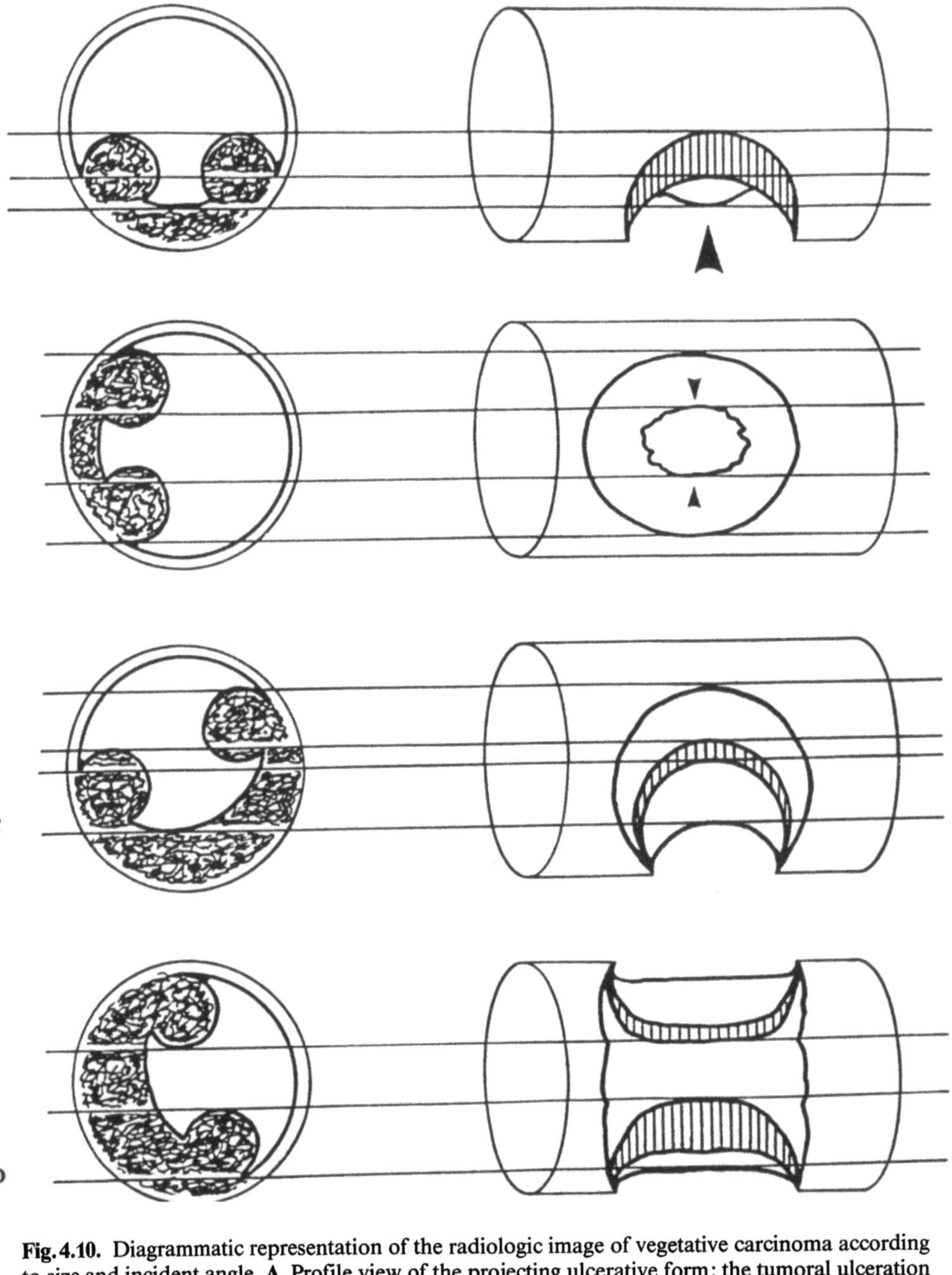

Fig. 4.10. Diagrammatic representation of the radiologic image of vegetative carcinoma according to size and incident angle. **A,** Profile view of the projecting ulcerative form: the tumoral ulceration is sometimes seen as a line with its concavity toward the lumen *(arrow)*. **B,** Frontally, the ulceration may be recognized by its outlines if they are distinct. The tumoral rim then appears well underlined. **C,** Three-quarter view: the complex image corresponds to the crescent or quarter of an orange appearance. **D,** The lesion extends over more than half the circumference, indenting the colonic margins. With certain incident angles it has a stenosing appearance despite the fact that there is no circumferential spread

ture of the ulceration, which is better seen radiologically than in the resected specimen.

4.3.2.1 Noncircumferential Vegetative Ulcerative Forms

In frontal view, the lesion is represented by the image of the tumoral outlines (usually irregular) in the intermarginal aspect. The image is obtained either by capillary attraction or the tangent effect, or as a filling defect in the pool (Figs. 4.11-14). As already mentioned, the ulceration is often difficult to show, particularly in this view. It may appear as an addition image within a filling defect (Fig. 4.11) or as a ring shadow bordering the inner side of the tumoral rim (Fig. 4.10 B). In this case, however, it cannot be distinguished from a more prominent part of the tumoral formation.

In profile or from three-quarter view, the image corresponds to the classic contour defect of single contrast. It looks more like a crescent in strict profile (Figs. 4.10, 13, 14). Most often, it is the image of a quarter of an orange which is obtained (Fig. 4.14). This is formed by the superimposition of the lesion's implantation limits circumferentially and the tumoral outlines tangential to the incident beam. The greater the lesion's circumferential spread, the deeper the indentation and the more typical the lesion's appearance (even more so when the infiltration and retraction accentuate the appearance of indentation). If the circumferential spread is greater than half the circumference, the indentation may affect both colonic borders from a frontal view but appear only on one side in a profile view (Fig. 4.13). The ulceration is only sometimes visible. In profile or from a three-quarter view, it is represented by the outwardly convex appearance of the lesion's external border (Fig. 4.15) or by an addition image ringed by the tumoral rim (Fig. 4.16).

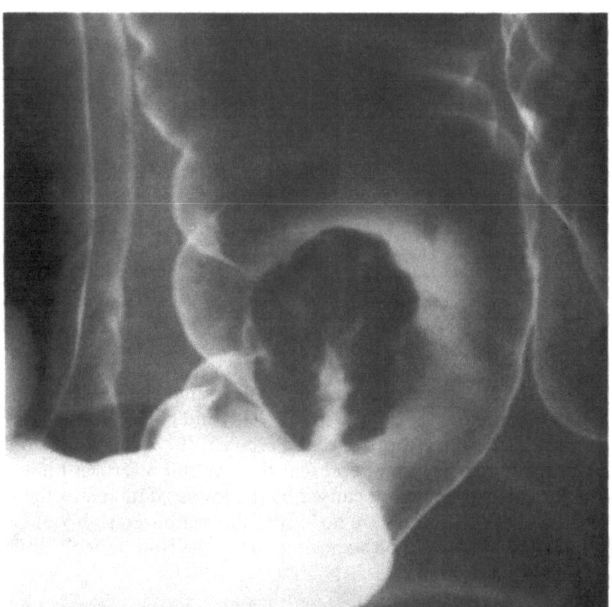

Fig. 4.11. Vegetative ulcerative carcinoma seen frontally. The tumoral contours are underlined by the pool. The ulceration appears as an addition image within a lacunar image

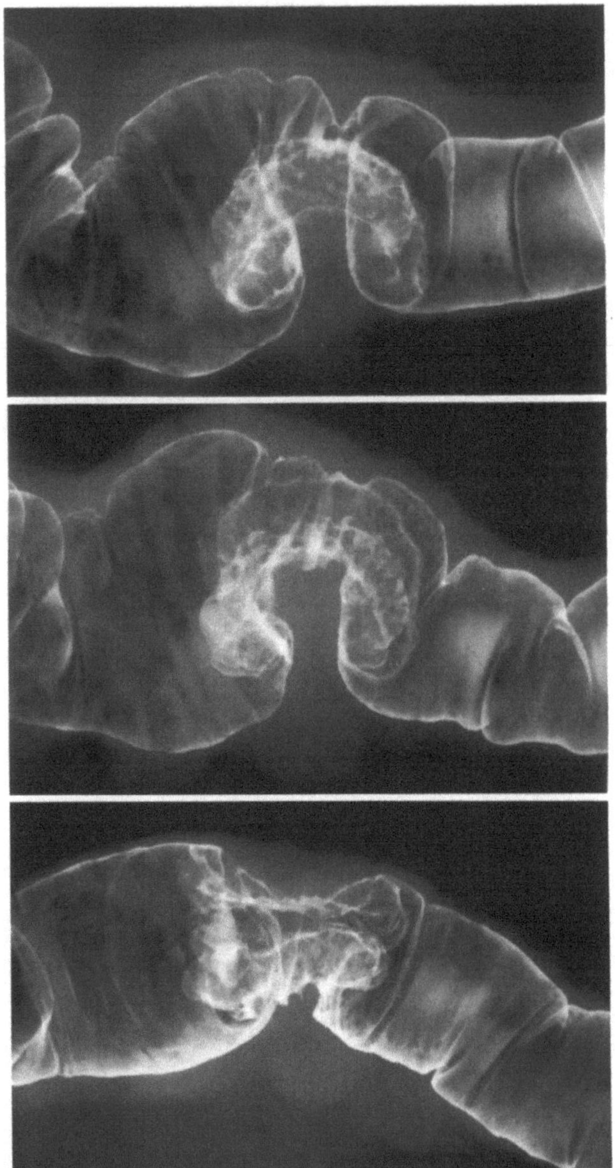

1

2

3

Fig. 4.13. Profile, three-quarter view, and frontal radiographs **(1, 2, 3)** of an anatomic example of ulcerative carcinoma (example in Fig. 4.12) and corresponding diagrammatic representation.
1 In profile, the upper border of the crescent **(b)** corresponds to the protruding part of the tumor. The lower border **(a)** may represent the parietal insertion limits or the bottom of the ulceration. Note the parietal retraction caused by the lesion: it increases the indentation **(c)**. **2** In three-quarter view, the tumoral outlines are no longer superimposed **(b-b')** and a crescent image forms. **3** Frontally, the lesion appears to be stenosing due to the simultaneous indentation of both margins. The ulceration is not evident

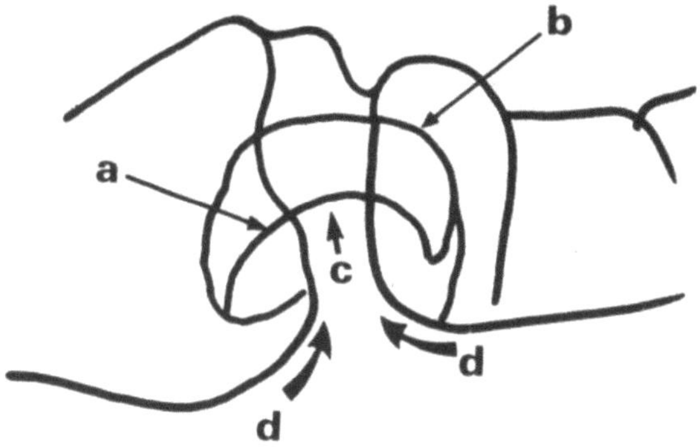

1

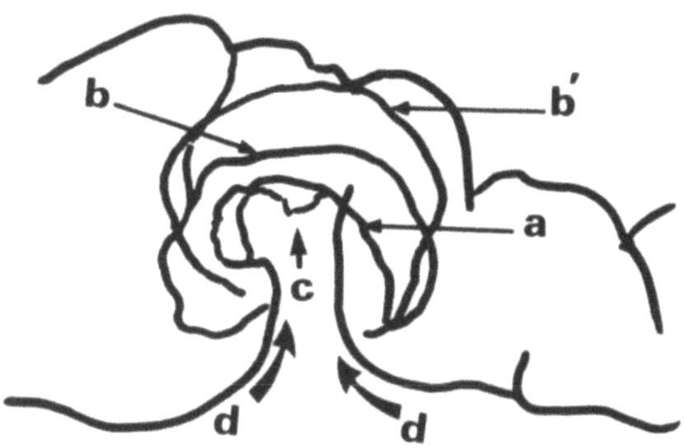

2

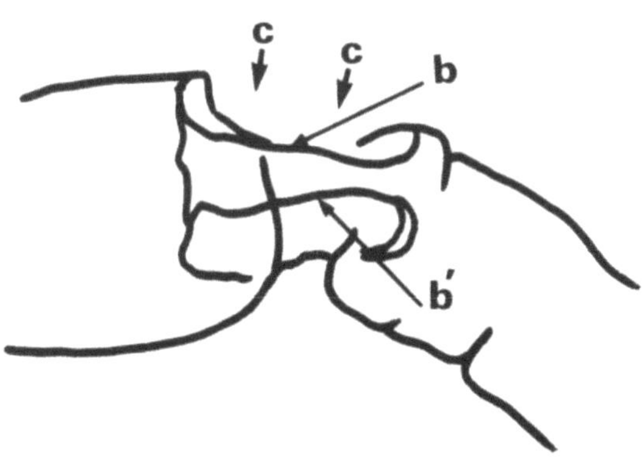

3

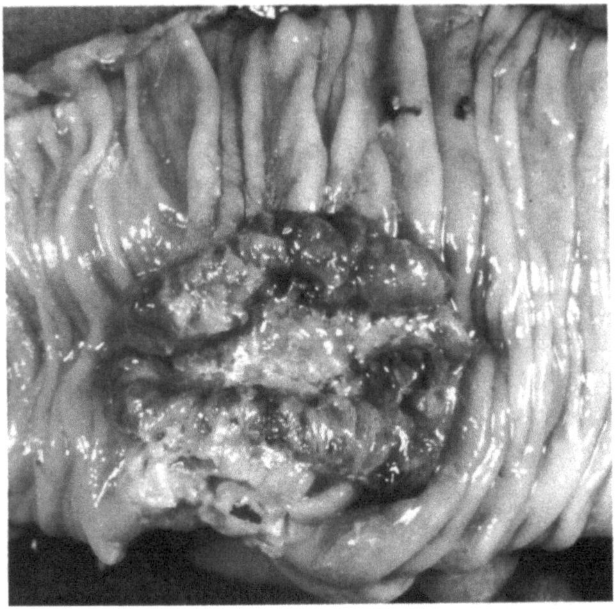

Fig. 4.12. Vegetative ulcerative carcinoma (anatomic example): the ulceration forms a large gully in the lesion

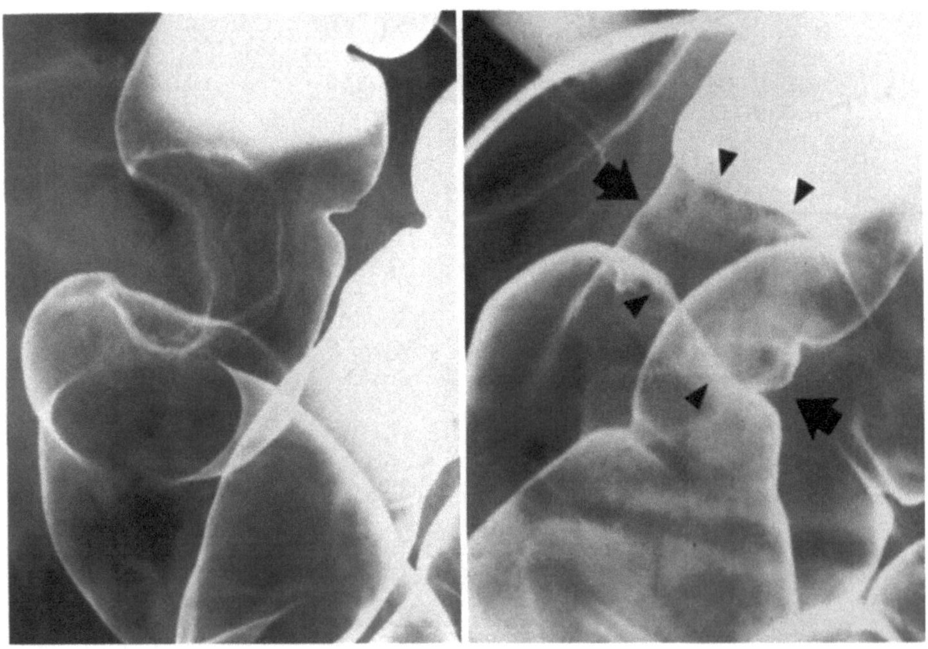

A B

Fig. 4.14. Noncircumferential vegetative ulcerative carcinoma. **A** Profile, crescent image. The ulceration is not evident. **B** Frontal view; only retraction of the colonic margins *(large arrows)* draws our attention. The pool emphasizes the proximal part of the lesion

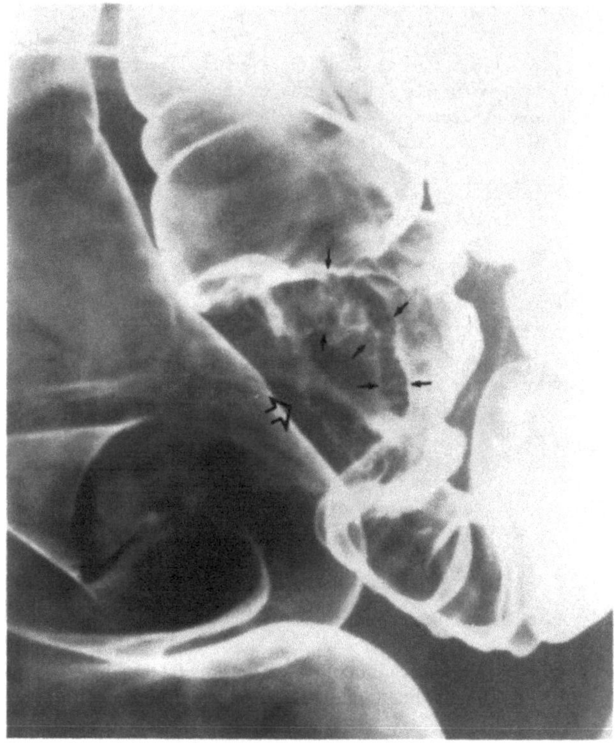

Fig. 4.15. Three-quarter view of vegetative ulcerative carcinoma. The ulceration is confirmed by the outward convexity of the external border of the crescent image *(open arrow)*. The tumoral rim is clearly defined

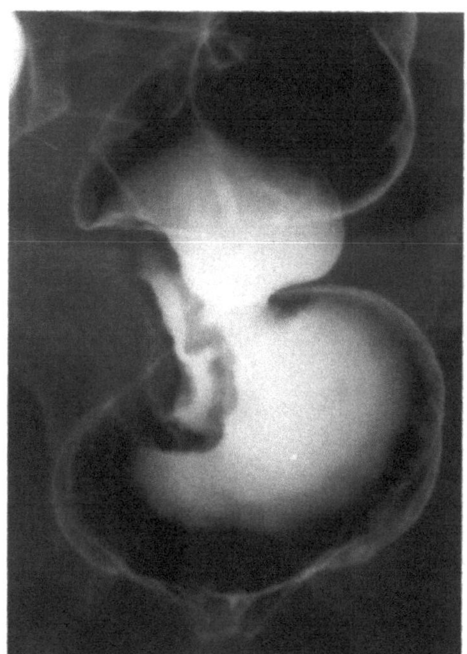

Fig. 4.16. Three-quarter view of vegetative ulcerative carcinoma. The ulceration appears to be filled with barium and ringed by the tumoral rim

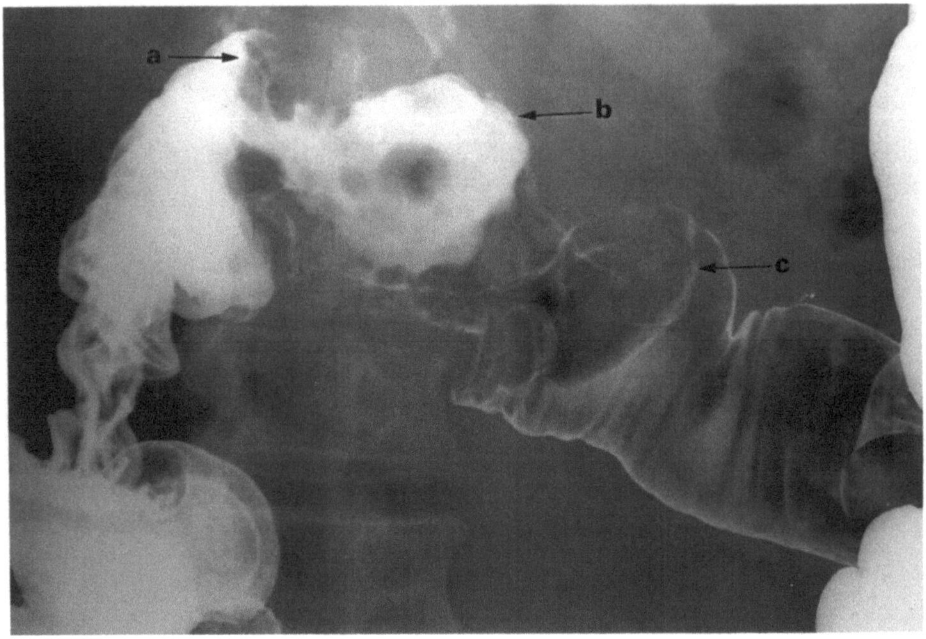

Fig. 4.17. Vegetative ulcerative carcinoma (stenosing). The tumoral poles are visualized in **a** by barium and in **c** by the tangent effect. The central ulceration **(b)** is large

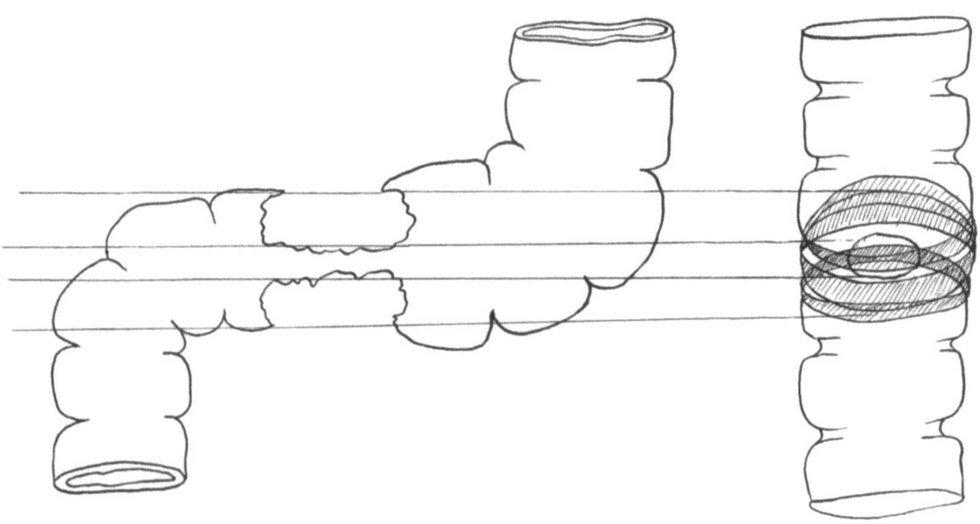

Fig. 4.18. Vegetative ulcerative carcinoma (stenosing). It is difficult to recognize tumoral stenosis in a frontal view

4.3.2.2 Circumferential Forms

Here we find the classic appearance or the ulcerated tumoral stenosis stretched between two tumoral poles (Fig. 4.17). Other than the classic "overhanging margin" and "shouldering" images seen in double contrast or those due to the pool sign (Fig. 4.17), certain appearances should be emphasized. These are related to the presence of misleading superimpositions masking the parietal indentation or, when the tumoral pole and stenosis are viewed frontally (incident beam is parallel to the stenosis) (Fig. 4.18). In these cases, the filling defect is missing and it is the demonstration of abnormal and unexplained lines which leads to the lesion's discovery. *Any unexplained longitudinal line corresponds to tumoral stenosis until proven otherwise* (Fig. 4.19). In cases of complete stenosis the barium column is blocked at the distal tumoral pole (10% of stenosing cancers). This pole, which forms a puffed invagination, is highly indicative, particularly if it is irregular and contains the beginning of tumoral stenosis at its center (Fig. 4.20). If there is any doubt with localized spasm, glucagon is injected intravenously. Nonopacification of the stenosis requires a second examination using water-soluble contrast media perorally or perrectally. This possibility is rare, however.

4.3.3 Strict Infiltrating Forms

According to Morson [6] strict infiltrating forms are rare. They result in a loss of expansibility for the colonic segment in question. The segment is rigid but the mucosa appears normal. If tumoral nodules are present the diagnosis is greatly facilitated.

4.4 Effectiveness of the Double Contrast Enema in Colorectal Carcinoma

Other than making possible early diagnosis and prevention of cancer, the double contrast technique enables simultaneous checks to be made for other colonic localizations of the tumoral process or associated polyps. We have found the association polyp-carcinoma in 52% of our cases and synchronous carcinoma in 8% of our cases. This in itself justifies a preoperative double contrast enema for all polyps or carcinoma discovered by other techniques.

Some claim that the double contrast enema misses colorectal carcinomas. A study by Kelvin's group [5] made it possible to assess this argument precisely. During a 5-year period, this author found 31 cases of unrecognized colorectal carcinoma (in six institutions). The error was purely perceptive in 52%, perceptive and due to technical failure in 32%, and due to interpretational error in 6% of the cases. For only 10% of lesions, which could not be seen retrospectively, was technical failure responsible. The authors estimate the percentage error for double contrast enema to be 1% (2 unrecognized colorectal carcinomas out of 197 cases). Among the different technical failures that can arise the author cites excess barium, insufficient distention, and film overexposure. He concludes (and we can only but emphasize this): "Radiologists must become familiar with

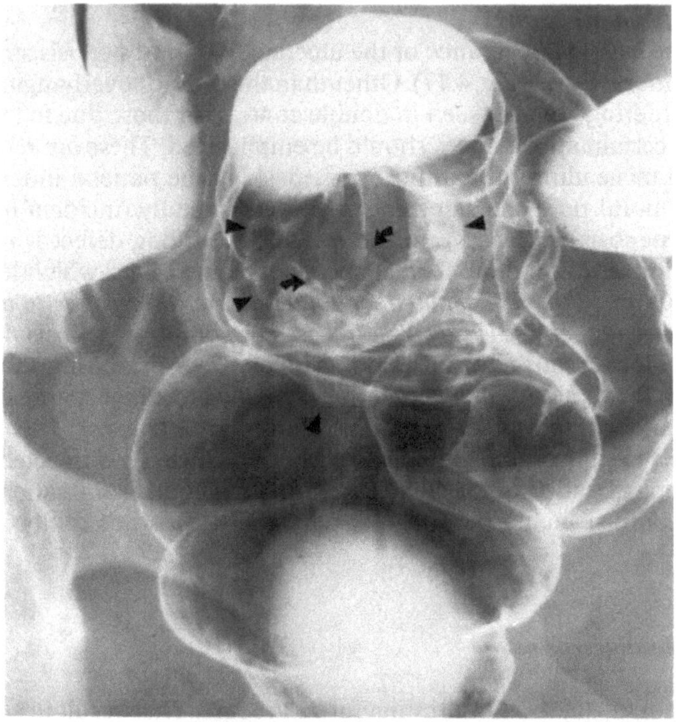

4.19 A

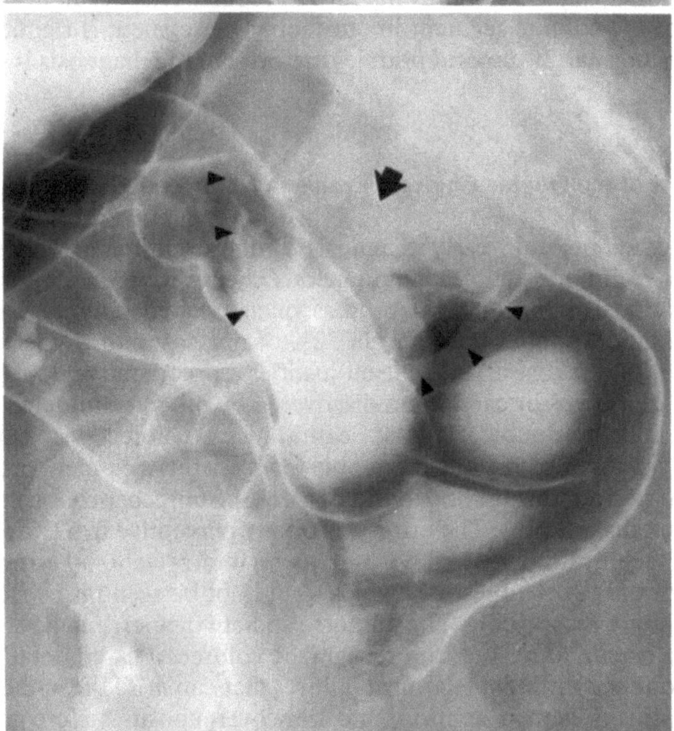

4.19 B

the principles of interpretation of lesions seen on double contrast studies, if the full value of the technique is to be realized."

Fig. 4.20. Stenosing carcinoma of the hepatic flexure. **a,** puffed tumoral protrusion in the lumen; **b,** beginnings of tumoral stenosis

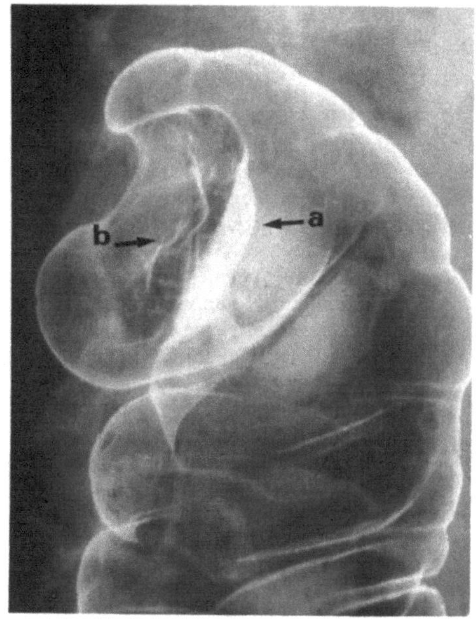

◁ **Fig. 4.19.** Vegetative ulcerative carcinoma (stenosing). **A** Frontal radiograph. This large tumoral lesion is seen frontally and is indicated only by the presence of abnormal lines, designating a tumoral pole *(arrowheads);* the stenosis is particularly indicated by the disappearance of the normal rectosigmoid contours *(curved arrows).* **B** In profile, the tumoral poles are shown by the tangent effect *(small arrows)* and tumoral stenosis appears *(large arrow)*

References

1. Ament AE, Alfidi RJ, Sridharrag P (1982) Basal indentation of sessile polypoïd lesions: a function of geometry rather than a sign of malignancy. Radiology 143: 341-344
2. Ekelund G, Lindstrom C, Rosengren JE (1974) Appearance and growth of early carcinoma of the colon and rectum. Acta Radiol 15: 670-679
3. Fenoglio CM, Nathan L (1973) The anatomic precursor of colorectal carcinoma. JAMA 231: 640
4. Figiel LS, Figiel SJ, Wietersen FK (1965) Roentgenologic observations of growth rates of colonic polyps and carcinoma. Acta Radiol 13: 417-429
5. Kelvin FM, Gardiner R, Vas W, Stevenson GW (1981) Colorectal carcinoma missed on double contrast barium enema study: a problem in perception. Am J Radiol 137: 307-313
6. Morson BC, Dawson IMP (1979) Gastrointestinal pathology. 2 nd edn. Blackwell, Oxford pp 648-680
7. Morson BC (1976) Genesis of colorectal cancer. Clinics Gastroenterol 5: 505-525
8. Potet F, Soullard J, Lambling A (1962) Polypes et cancers du rectosigmoïde, étude critique de la notion de dégénérescence et hypothèse de filiation. Presse Med 70: 865-868
9. Soullard J, Potet F (1975) La prévention des cancers recto coliques. Arch Fr Mal App Dig 64: 197-200
10. Weissman A, Grellet J (1977) Rôle prépondérant du radiologiste dans la prévention du cancer rectocolique par le dépistage des polypes. J Radiol Electrol 58: 193-198
11. Weissman A, Riche MC, Clot M, Grellet J (1978) Intérêt du lavement en double contraste (mucographie) dans le bilan pré opératoire du cancer rectocolique (résultats préliminaires). Journées Francophones de Gastroentérologie - jan 1978 - Paris
12. Welin S, Welin G (1976) The double contrast examination of the colon. Experiences with the Welin modifications. Thieme, Stuttgart

5 Villomas

For Morson [1] regard villomas are a simple form of "adenoma" (villous adenoma). If this were the case, it would make sense to study them in the chapter on polyps. Nevertheless, internists traditionally exclude them from this category in light of their macroscopic appearance which poses particular diagnostic and therapeutic problems.

According to Soullard, villomas make up 10% of benign colonic tumors. They are mainly located in the rectosigmoid (85%-95%) and have a high degree of malignant change which varies, according to author, from 38,5% to 90%. Macroscopically, these tumors may appear as common sessile or pedunculated polyps. Most often, they are sessile, spread out on the surface and may become quite large. They may appear as a carpet-like tumor which protrudes only slightly but may extend circumferentially. Two groups can be determined among the different radiologic appearances: (1) nonspecific and (2) indicative or even specific features.

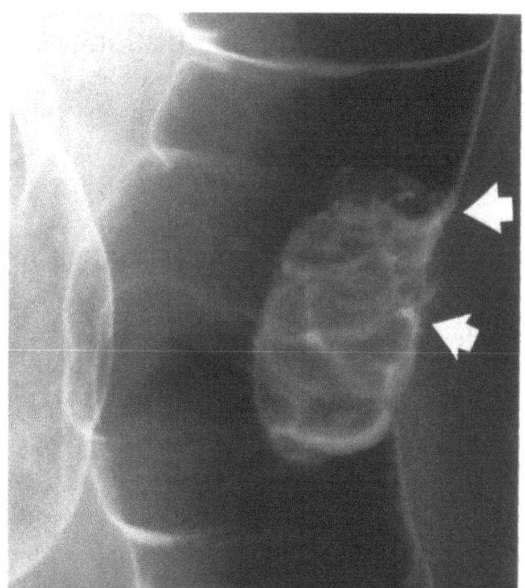

Fig. 5.1. "Intermediate polyp" type villoma with polycyclic contours and areolar surface. This appearance is nonspecific

5.1 Nonspecific Features

These are of sessile, intermediate, or pedunculated polyps where nothing on the radiograph suggests their villous nature. Their size may vary from several millimeters to several centimeters and they may have regular contours. Polycyclic contours and an areolar surface (Fig. 5.1) are classically considered to be indicative but not specific since polyadenomas may have a similar appearance.

5.2 Indicative and Specific Features

Two features seem to have a certain indicative value: (1) large volume of a strictly vegetative tumor that appears noninfiltrated and (2) carpet-like proliferation.

1. The large volume is not in itself pathognomonic, but a strictly nonulcerated lesion greater than 4–5 cm is, in principle, a villoma. A certain number of signs may support this hypothesis: the large basal indentation; the "hairy" aspect of the contours due to the villous fungosities; dense patches of barium flocculation on the tumoral surface caused by abundant mucus secretion (Fig. 5.2); and modification of the form of the vegetative lesion during the examination. This is due to the particularly soft nature of the tumor (Fig. 5.3), unlike the rigid character of advanced carcinoma

2. The "carpet-like" aspect of the tumor is equally characteristic. The tumor spread is fairly large. Seen frontally, the tumor has a spongy, areolar appearance due to the seepage of barium between the villosity bundles (Figs. 5.4, 5.5). Often early stages of flocculation with a pinpoint appearance can be seen. The borders of the tumor, which generally has vague contours, may be clearly outlined in the intermarginal aspect if the lesion is sufficiently raised. They will be less so if the tumor is flat.

The tumor is demonstrated at the colonic margin by an interruption of this line, which becomes irregular, broken, or blurred. The lesion still causes an indentation, which is usually minor, however, since the tumor is only slightly raised ("bas-relief" tumor) (Fig. 5.6). Discovery of these localized abnormalities in the double contrast study should first suggest a diagnosis of carpet-like villous lesion before one of poor preparation or segmentary colitis (postinflammatory polyposis).

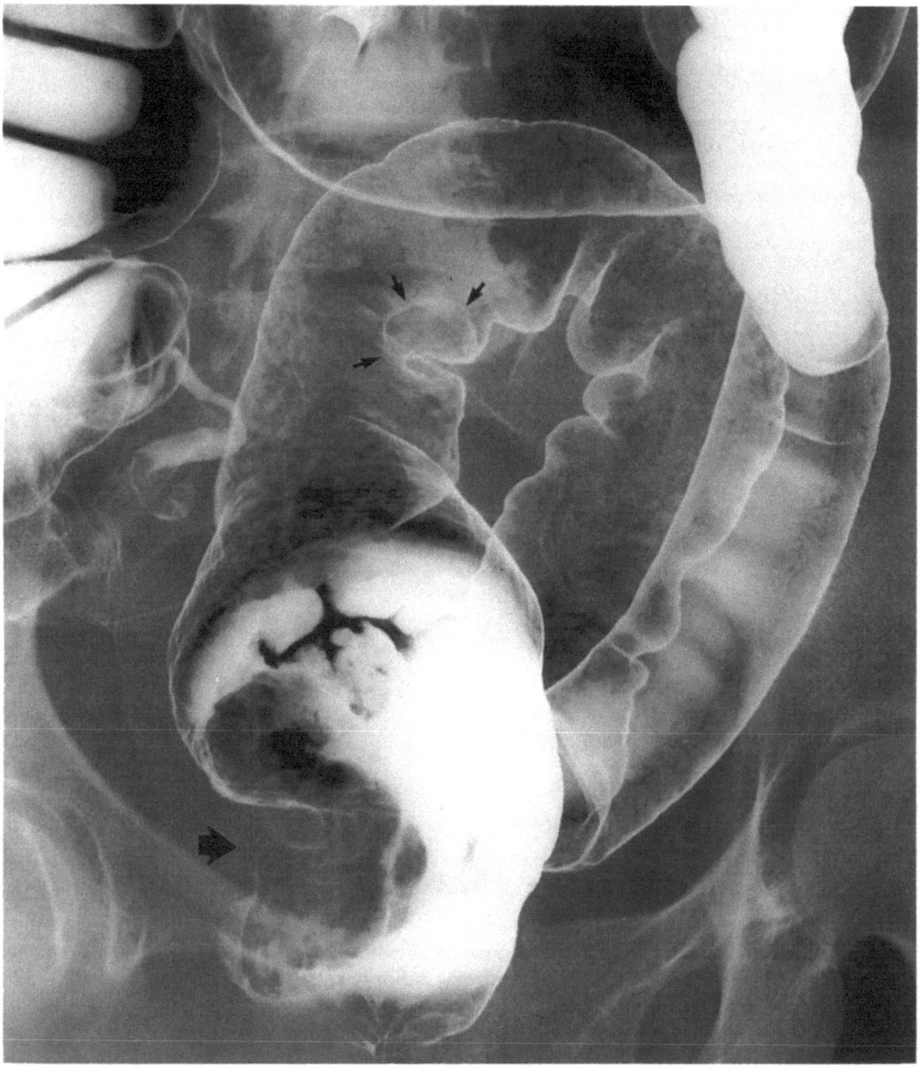

A

Fig. 5.2. Large villoma with severe dysplasia associated with sigmoid cancer 1,5 cm in diameter *(small arrows)*. **A,** Frontal view: indentation in the right rectal wall; polycyclic lacuna; patchy appearance of the barium, which penetrates between the fungosities. **B,** see page 106

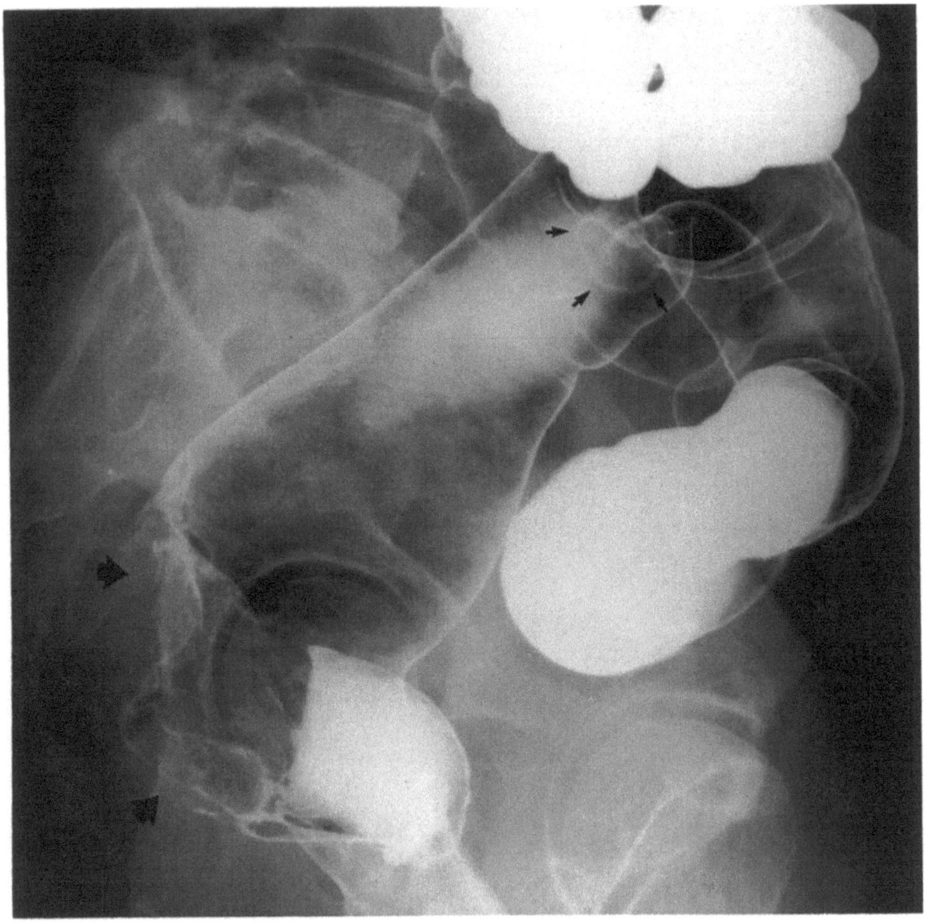

B

Fig. 5.2. Large villoma with severe dysplasia associated with sigmoid cancer 1,5 cm diameter (small arrows) **B,** profile view: indentation of the entire posterior rectal wall

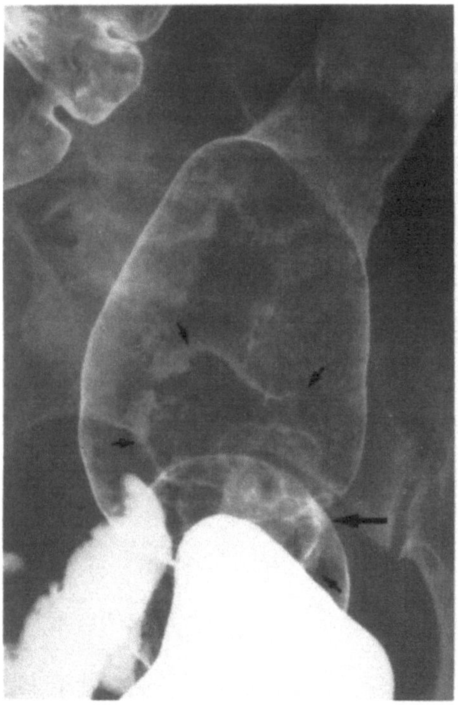

A

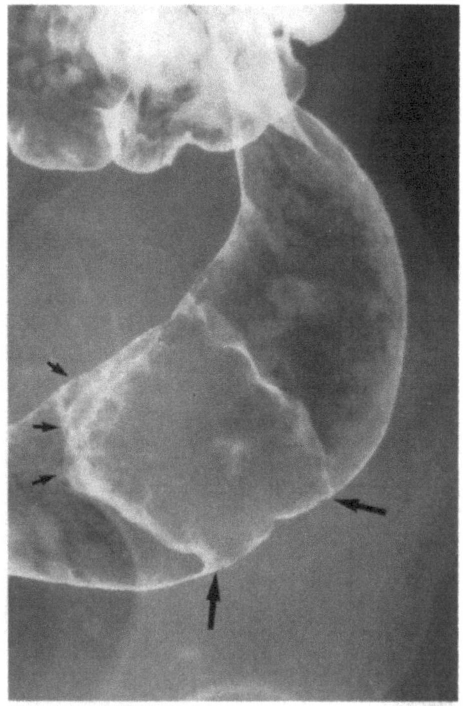

B

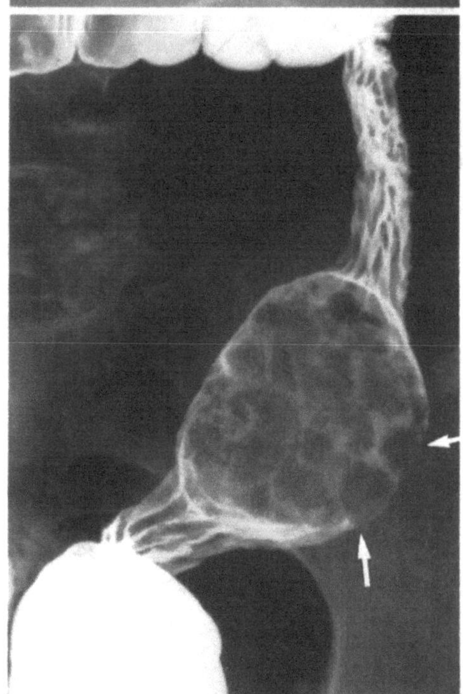

C

Fig. 5.3. Sessile villoma with relatively narrow base (base is designated by *large arrows*). **A** The lesion is partially visible in the pool. It has irregular contours. **B** Change in form - trabecular appearance particularly at the top *(small arrows)*. **C** New change in form with spasm during the same radiological examination. It has a distinct alveolar, spongy appearance. The narrow base is clearly visible

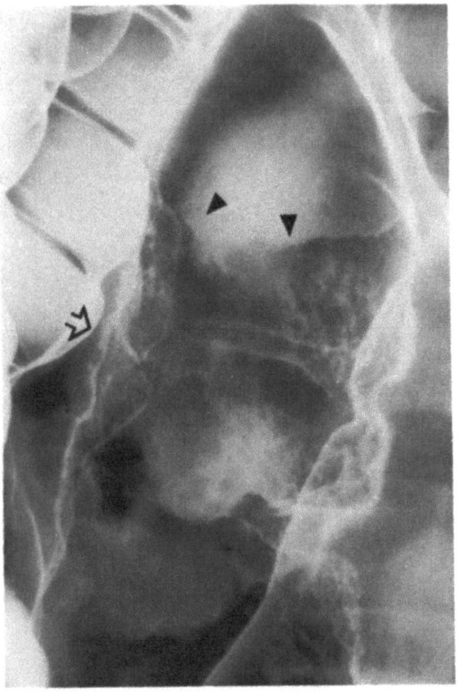

Fig. 5.4. Circumferential carpet-like villous lesion of the sigmoid colon. Note the blurry aspect of the borders, the slight indentation *(open arrow)*, the spongy appearance of the colonic mucosa, and the clear limitation of the tumoral pole *(arrows)*. (Courtesy of Dr. Mombet, Paris)

5.3 The Radiologic Diagnosis of Malignancy Remains Problematic

Welin [4] interpreted the presence of a basal indentation as negative sign since (cf. Chap 4), they found this in all villous lesions with invasive cancer and not in benign lesions. We consider the indentation to be independent of the problem of malignant change, even though it is more frequently found in more advanced lesions. Ulceration of a tumor is certainly a better indicator. In this case, however, the tumor already corresponds to advanced vegetative ulcerative carcinoma. In any case, only a histologic examination will confirm the benign or malignant nature of the tumor. It is, nevertheless, important that a diagnosis of villoma be considered and confirmed histologically prior to surgery so that a limited operation such as mucosectomy can be suggested. This therapeutic strategy is fundamental, especially for rectal tumors, since it avoids abdominal-perineal resections.

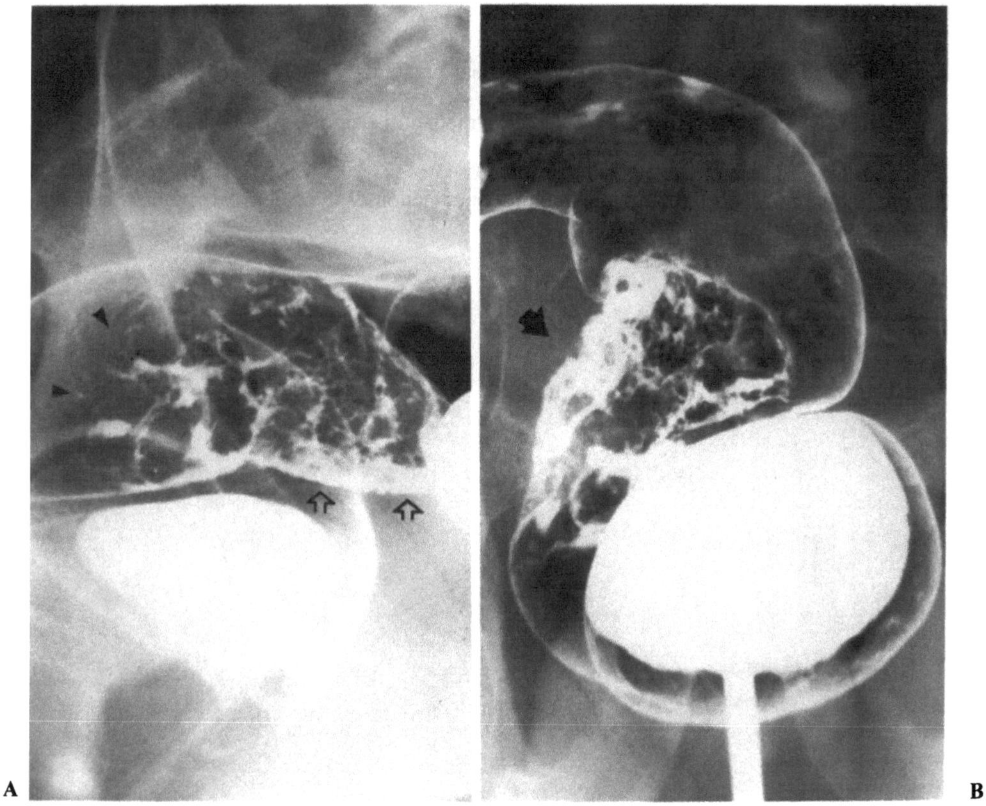

Fig. 5.5. Noncircumferential carpet-like villoma of the rectum: **A,** note the areolar relief of the lesion, the absence of distinct limits *(black arrows),* and the slight degree of indentation *(open arrow);* **B,** note the more distinct indentation

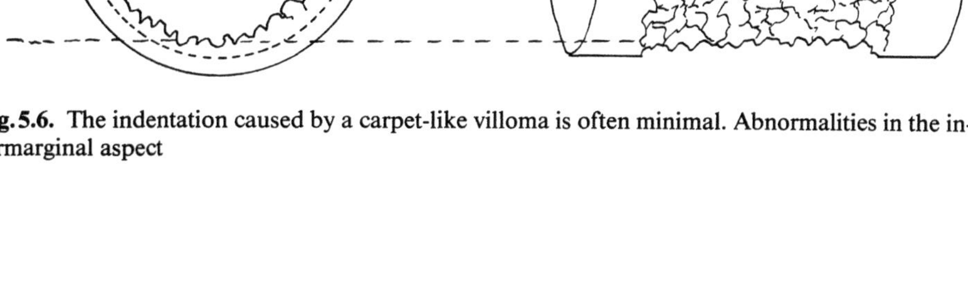

Fig. 5.6. The indentation caused by a carpet-like villoma is often minimal. Abnormalities in the intermarginal aspect

References

1. Morson BC, Dawson IMP (1979) Gastrointestinal pathology. 2nd edn. Blackwell, Oxford pp 686-704
2. Potet F, Soullard J (1973) Anatomopathologie et modalités évolutives spontanées des polypes et polyposes coliques. Rev Prat 23: 2219-2235
3. Soullard J (1975) Proctologie. Masson, Paris p 399
4. Welin S, Welin G (1976) The double contrast examination of the colon. Experiences with the Welin modification. Thieme, Stuttgart

6 Ulcerative Colitis

Double contrast represents a considerable advance for the diagnosis of colitis. It makes possible the detection of early signs, diagnosis of the etiology with a good margin of security, and clear definition of the limits of the disease's extension. Inflammatory colitis is above all a disease of the colonic mucosa. Its early diagnosis depends on the evaluation of indirect signs and especially on direct evidence of the mucosal injury shown by double contrast.

Several studies attest to the reliability of the double contrast enema concerning ulcerative colitis [2-6]. According to Laufer [3], endoscopic correlation is good in 95% of cases. Suspicion of inflammatory colitis may necessitate a change in patient preparation: laxatives and purgatives may be reduced or omitted, for the ambulatory patient; cleansing enemas may be reduced or omitted; and the low-residue diet is maintained. The examination is contraindicated if toxic megacolon is suspected. Otherwise, the risk is no greater than for a barium enema as long as insufflation is carefully performed. It is often better tolerated [3].

6.1 Radiologic Pathology

The radiologic appearance of ulcerative colitis is closely related to the severity of the lesions. A review of the major characteristics is necessary in order to facilitate interpretation of the images. Ulcerative colitis is primarily a disease of the mucosa. The rectum is almost always affected (as a rule, the first site of the disease). Also characteristic is the proximal extension (left to right). The mucosal lesions are continuous (uninterrupted) and involve the entire circumference of a given colonic segment. The appearance of the mucosa varies according to the severity of acute attacks, however, lesions at different stages may be found in different areas in the same patient.

Three endoscopic appearances can be described during acute attacks:

1. Early lesions give the mucosa, which bleeds when swabbed, a fragile, speckled, congested appearance. Macroscopic ulcerations cannot be detected.
2. At a more advanced stage, small disseminated ulcerations appear and the transversal folding of the mucosa disappears [5].
3. Severe lesions are represented by confluent ulcerations forming deep longitudinal gullies opposite the teniae. Only a few traces of mucosa remain. Pseudopolypoid patterns appear: islands of raised edematous mucosa surrounded by ulcerations; inflammatory granuloma (exuberant granulations); and digital

pseudopolyps or bridged polyps formed by mucous flaps partially detached from the submucous coat and reepithelialized.

The ulcerations regress during remission but the mucosa remains fragile and rarely returns to its normal state. Pseudopolypoid patterns of the mucous relief persist at least in part. Fibrosis of the submucous coat and hypertrophy of the muscular coat result in a shortening of the colon, depression of the flexures, narrowing of the caliber with the possibility of stenosis, and a loss of haustration.

6.2 Radiologic Appearance

In double contrast radiologic appearance is closely related to the state of the mucosa.

6.2.1 Motor Activity Changes and Caliber and Haustral Abnormalities

Motor activity changes, and caliber and haustral abnormalities (functional and/or organic) are detected as with the standard technique.

At the early stage, either during filling or after insufflation, nonspecific signs indicate mucous edema and hypertonia. These signs are represented by:

1. An unusual spastic contraction of a pathologic segment.
2. A flattening, squaring, or inversion of the haustra.
3. Loss of haustration in a colonic segment whose caliber is often narrowed (it should be remembered that loss of haustration is not necessarily pathologic in the left colon and may also occur without pathologic significance in the right colon. It is generally transitory and associated with a normal double contrast study).
4. Major evacuation of the enema at the end of the examination with thickening of mucous folds in the descending colon. These functional modifications generally regress along with the evolution of the disease.

At later stages:

1. Barium often runs through an atonic colon.
2. The caliber narrows, often symmetrically, creating a "lead pipe" tubulated appearance. Strictures which are sometimes asymmetric may appear (Fig. 6.1).
3. The overall length of the colon is reduced. The flexures are depressed.
4. The rectum is small; Houston's valves are obliterated; the postrectal space (measured opposite S_4) is widened; and the ampulla has a "spindle-like" appearance (Figs. 6.2, 6.3).
5. The ileocecal valve is dilated and incompetent (Fig. 6.4). These images may be definitive, representing the development of irreversible lesions. In any case they may vary greatly over a period of time, thus demonstrating their functional nature.

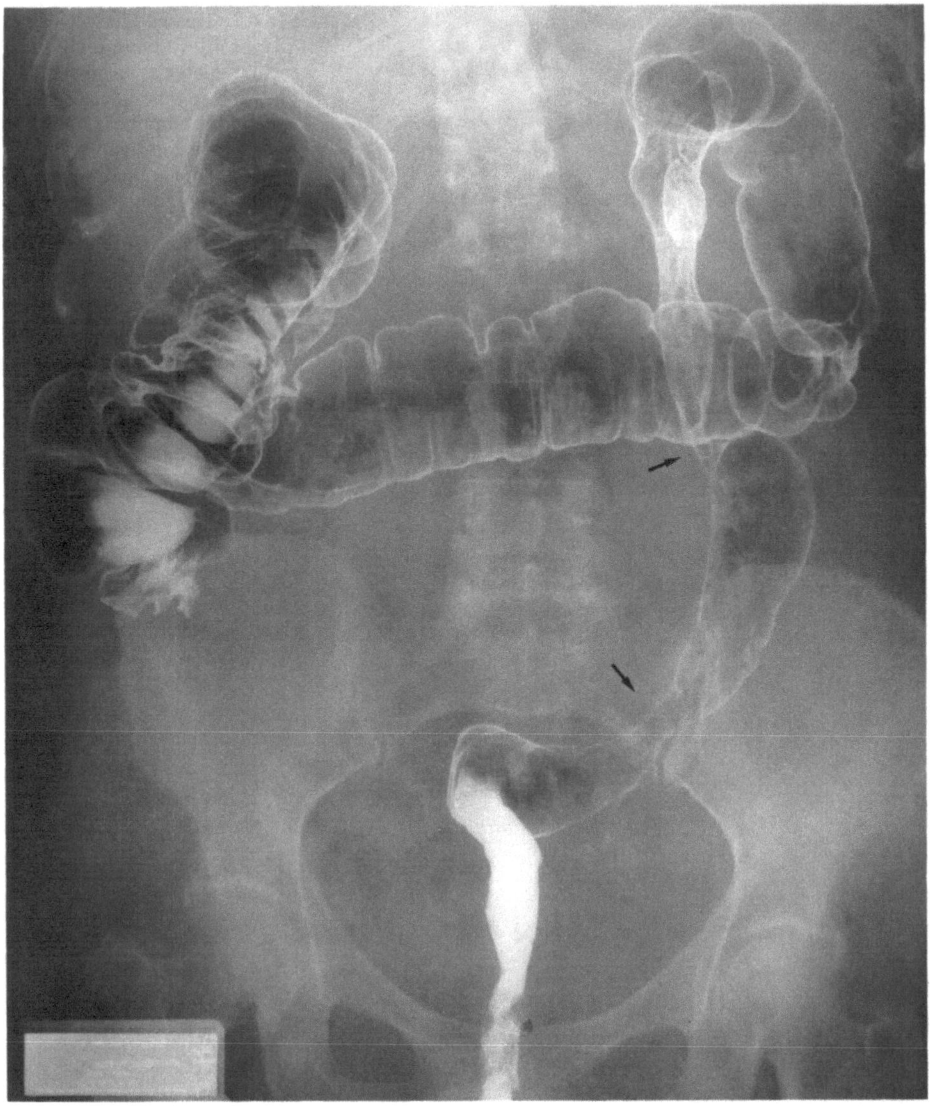

Fig. 6.1. Long-standing ulcerative colitis. Note the narrowing of the rectum and asymmetric stenosis throughout the sigmoid (rectracted) and descending colon. Caliber and haustra are normal in the transverse colon, but pseudopolyps indicate previous acute attacks

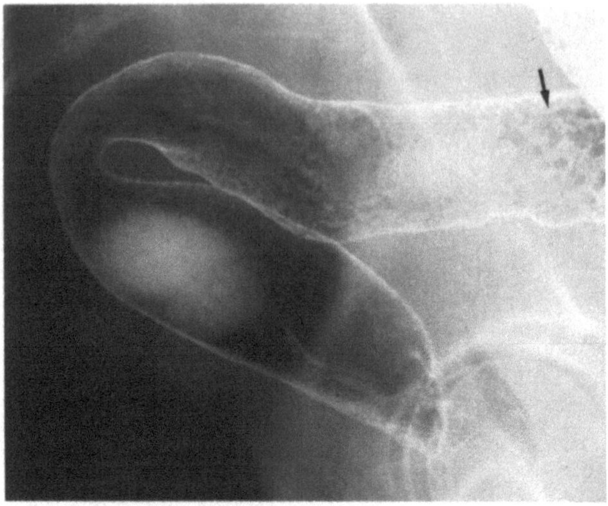

Fig. 6.2. Treated ulcerative colitis: profile radiograph of the rectum. Note the narrowed caliber and spindle-like appearance of the ampulla; obliteration of Houston's valves; and granular appearance of the image, showing pseudopolyps in the sigmoid colon *(arrow)*

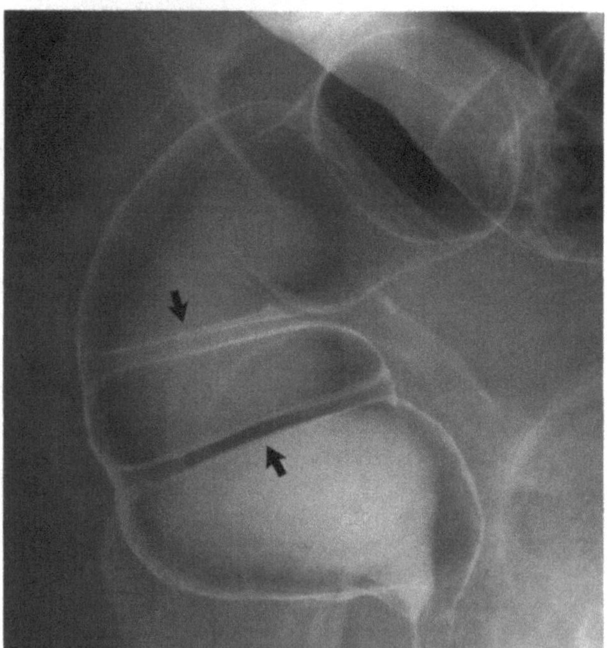

Fig. 6.3. Normal rectum. Note Houston's valves, which are clearly visible *(arrows)*, and distension of the ampulla

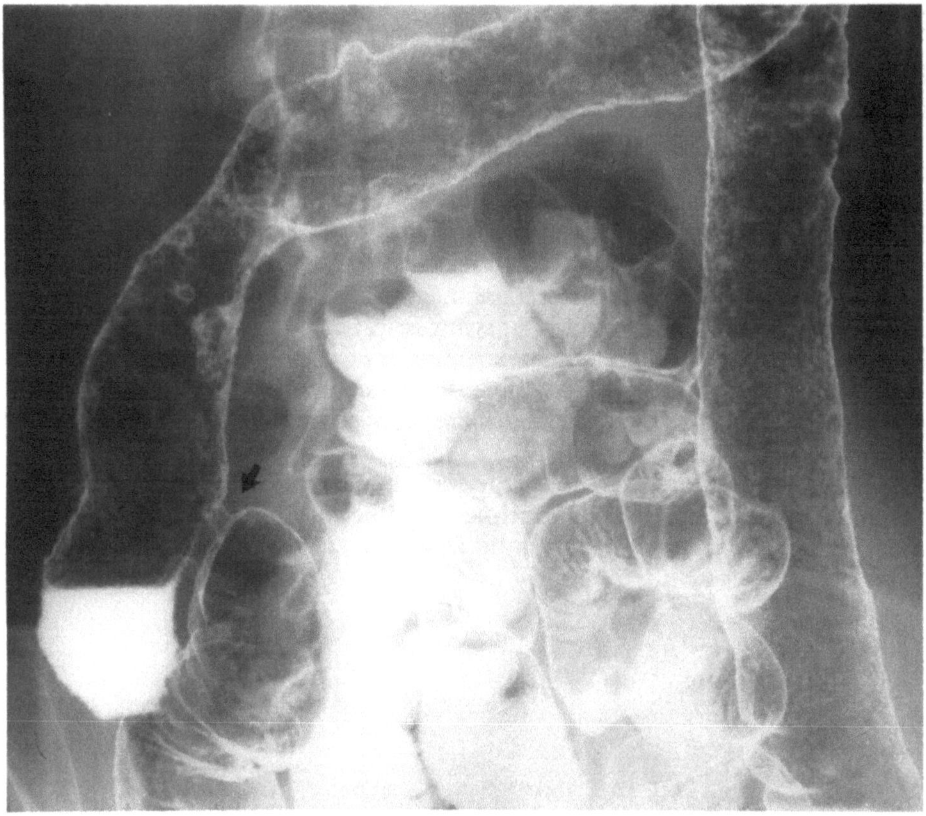

Fig. 6.4. Ulcerative colitis. Valvular dilatation *(arrow)* with massive reflux into the terminal ileum. The cecum and hepatic flexure are distinctly shortened and pseudopolyps indicate this is a long-standing affliction

6.2.2 *Changes in the Colonic Mucosa (Walls and Margins)*

Other than showing functional aspects and caliber changes, double contrast clearly demonstrates the state of the colonic mucosa. Three stages can be described. They correspond perfectly to endoscopic appearances and represent lesions of increasing severity. They may coexist in different colonic segments or appear successively during acute attacks.

Essential radiologic characteristics of these lesions are their continuity, absence of a normal zone in an affected segment, and relative regularity. This description is essential for the differential diagnosis of Crohn's disease, where the lesions are typically discontinuous, asymmetric, irregularly distributed, and associated with large parietal edema, creating transverse grooves which are absent in ulcerative colitis [8]. The three double contrast aspects of the colonic walls and margins during acute attack are: congestive, ulcerative, ulceroproliferous.

1. The congestive appearance is the earliest encountered. It represents a hyperemic, speckled mucosa without macroscopic ulceration. The double contrast radiograph taken frontally is heterogeneous: the juxtaposition of small

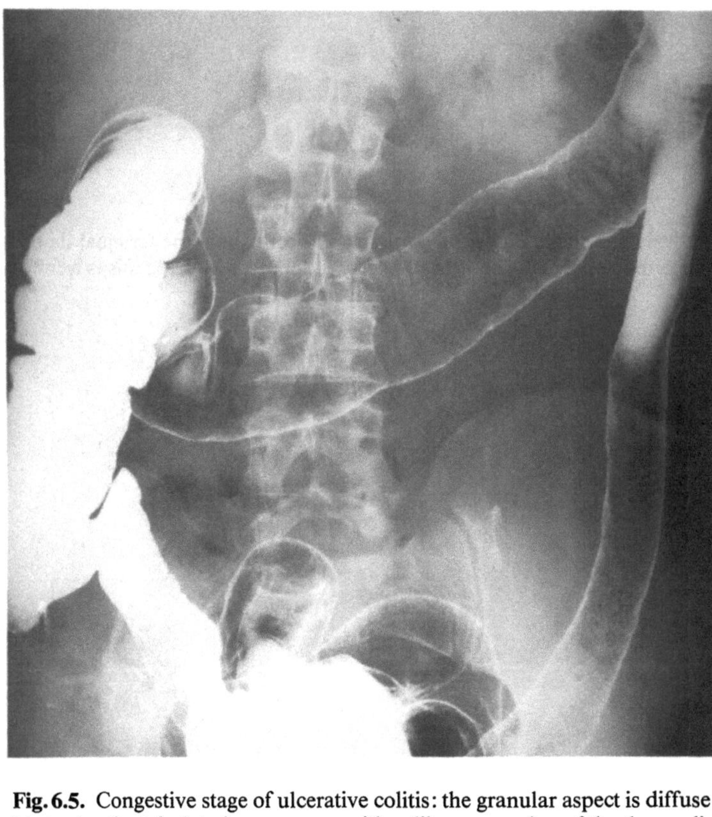

Fig. 6.5. Congestive stage of ulcerative colitis: the granular aspect is diffuse and relatively uniform. Note also the tubulated appearance with caliber narrowing of the descending colon and reflux into the terminal ileum

opaque and radiotransparent zones creates a highly indicative granular, areolar, and reticular image (Figs. 6.5, 6.6). The mucosal line becomes thickened and irregular. The thickness varies from millimeter to millimeter. These images cover the entire circumference of a given segment, are continuous and are homogeneously distributed. As a rule, there is a clear division between the diseased section and the rest of the bowel (Fig. 6.7). Diagnostic problems at this stage are easily resolved since the granular appearance is different from that in other cases where the double contrast image is also heterogeneous such as: microspiculation and cracking as discussed previously (see Chap. 2). The heterogeneity caused by fecal matter may sometimes be in question but is generally much coarser.

2. Ulcer formation represents a second stage: Frontally ulcers are indicated by the presence of multiple opaque spots variable in size and form sometimes encircled by a ring of edema (target image; Figs. 6.8, 6.9). In profile, they appear as notched margins and more shallow than in the standard technique. The density of these ulcerations varies and the surrounding mucosa is often granular.

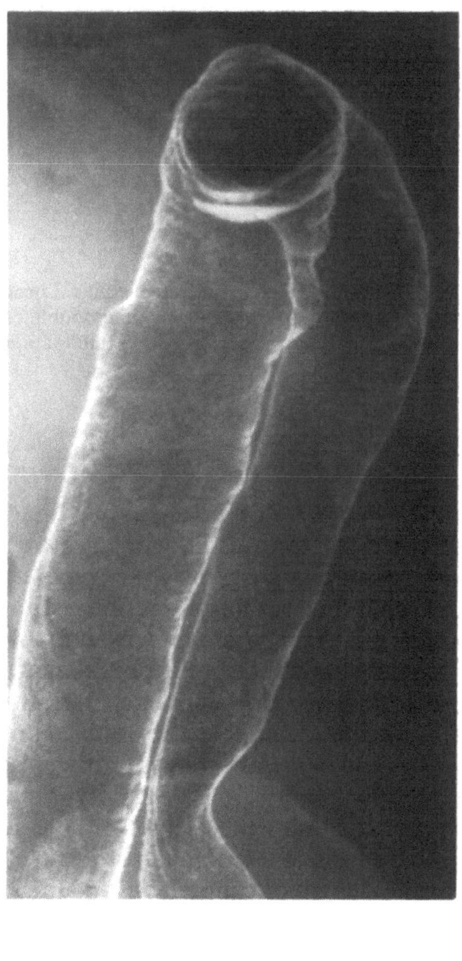

Fig. 6.6. Early stage of ulcerative colitis: margins are thickened and irregular. The walls have a granular appearance (endoscopically, the mucosa is fragile, hyperemic, and speckled without visible ulceration)

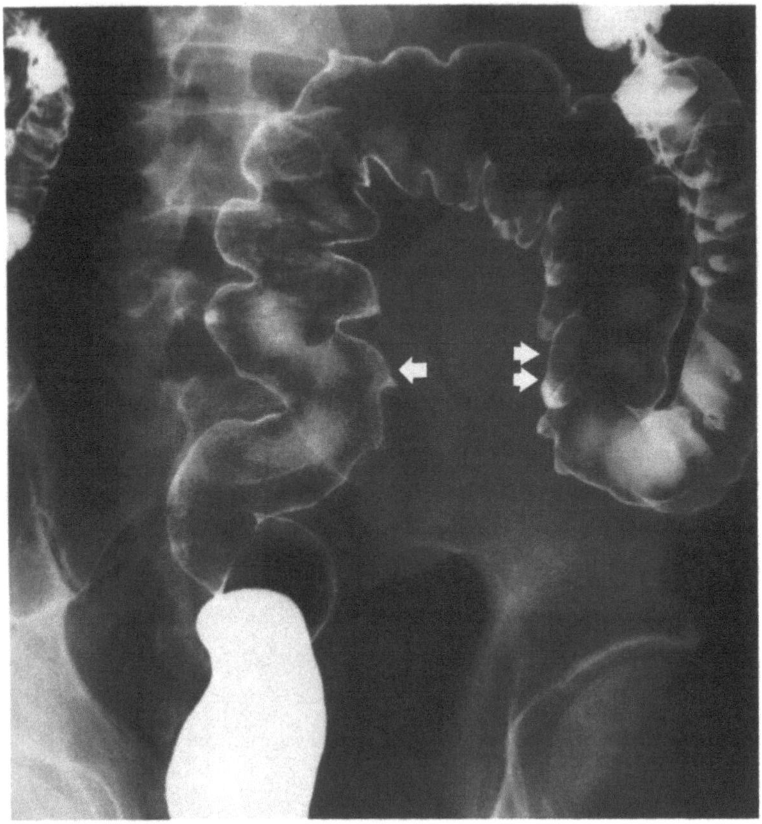

Fig. 6.7. Congestive stage ulcerative colitis. Localized form: the distal sigmoid has a reticular and granular appearance *(single arrow)*; the double contrast image of the proximal sigmoid is normal *(double arrow)*; haustral abnormalities (alternation) are due to coexisting diverticlculosis

3. When the ulcers deepen or join together and are associated with pseudo polypoid patterns, resulting images are more complex. In predominantly ulcerative forms opaque spots with irregular contours frontally, and double contour and collarbutton addition images in profile (T shape) are characteristic (Fig. 6.10). In predominantly pseudopolypoid forms, it is the filling defect either circled by barium or in the pool that is most frequently encountered (Fig. 6.11). Quite often pseudopolyps and ulcerations are associated (Fig. 6.12).

4. During remissions the double contrast image may return to normal. Only caliber and haustral changes or the presence of pseudopolyps indicate previous acute attack (Fig. 6.4). Pseudopolyps may be numerous, joined (Fig. 6.11) or disseminated, and regular (Fig. 6.13) or irregular (Fig. 6.14) in form. The differential diagnosis of adenomatous or other polyposis would only be in question if haustral length or caliber abnormalities were absent.

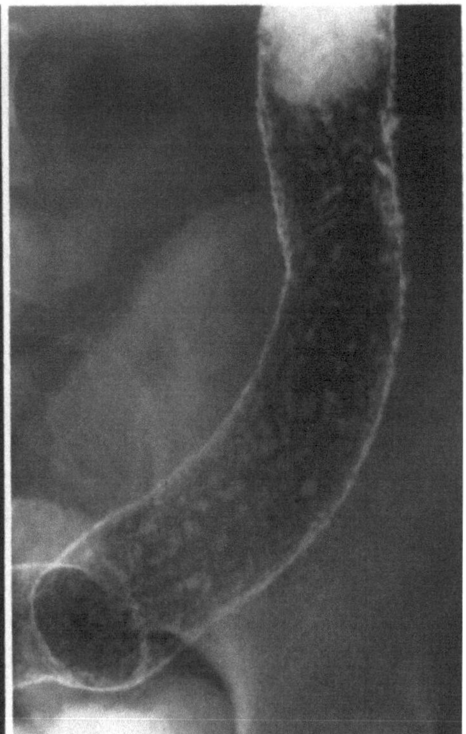

6.9

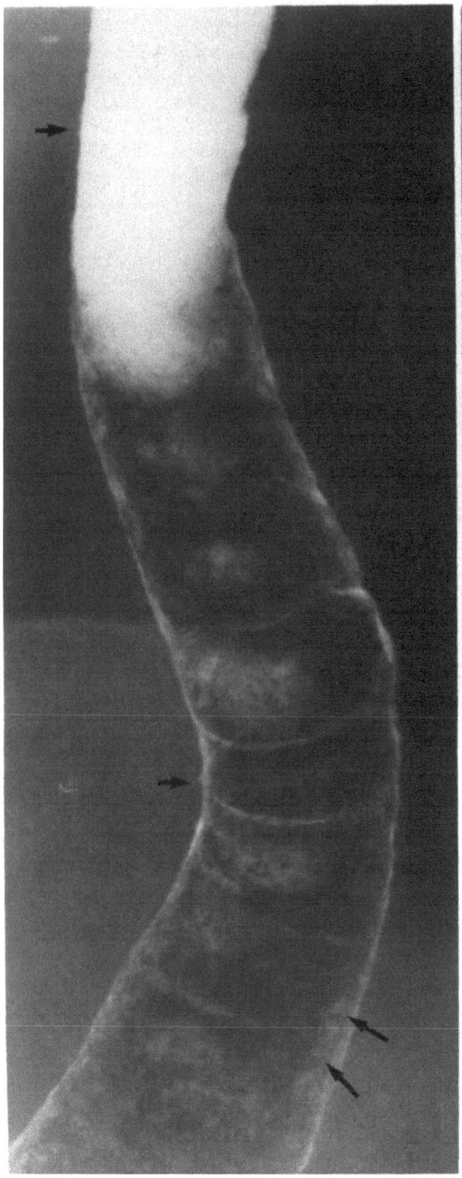

6.8

Fig. 6.8. Ulcerated form of ulcerative colitis. Opaque spots caused by ulcerations on the walls as well as borders appear on this heterogeneous double contrast image *(arrows)*

Fig. 6.9. Acute attack of ulcerative colitis. Ulcerated form. Ulcerations are greater in size and number than in the patient in Fig. 6.8

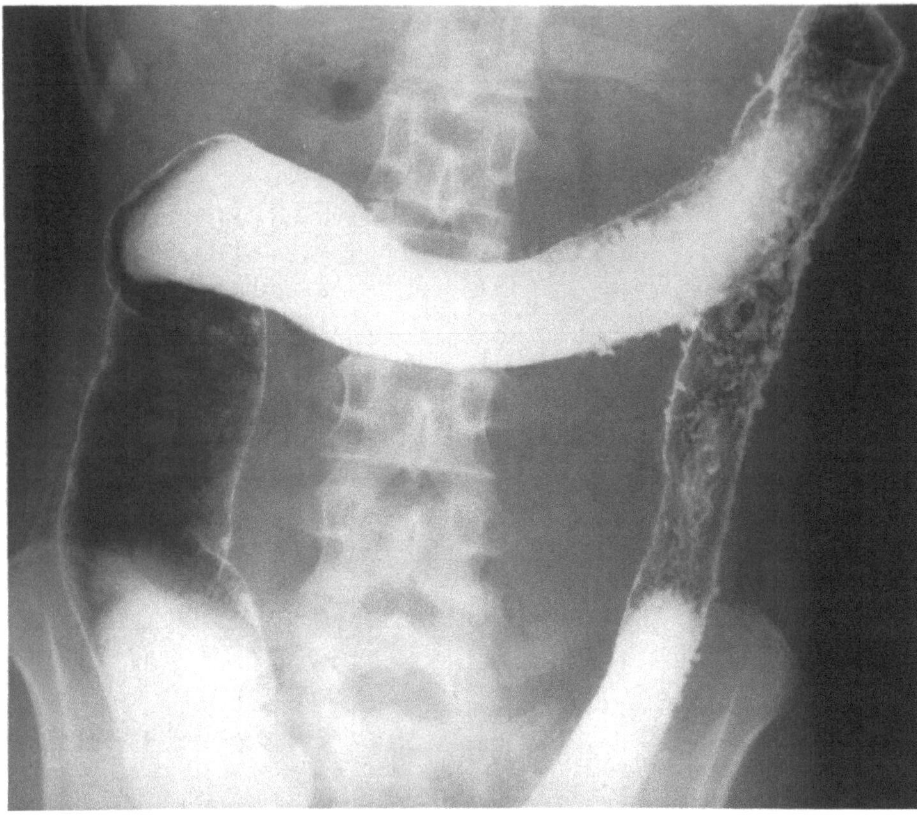

Fig. 6.10. Acute attack of ulcerative colitis. Ulcerated form: tubular aspect of the entire colon with loss of haustration. Narrowing of the left colon: *On the right* the double contrast image appears heterogeneous and *on the left* deep collar-button and thorn-like ulcerations are seen

Complications: Anal fistulae, while rarely associated with ulcerative colitis, may occur (Fig. 6.11). Toxic megacolon as already stated is a contraindication to all barium enemas. Carcinoma, especially in diffuse and long-standing forms, may be detected by double contrast, but endoscopy seems to us to be a more reliable method.

In conclusion, double contrast makes for a satisfactory exploration of ulcerative colitis. It provides important information for early diagnosis by its precise evaluation of the extent of the disease.

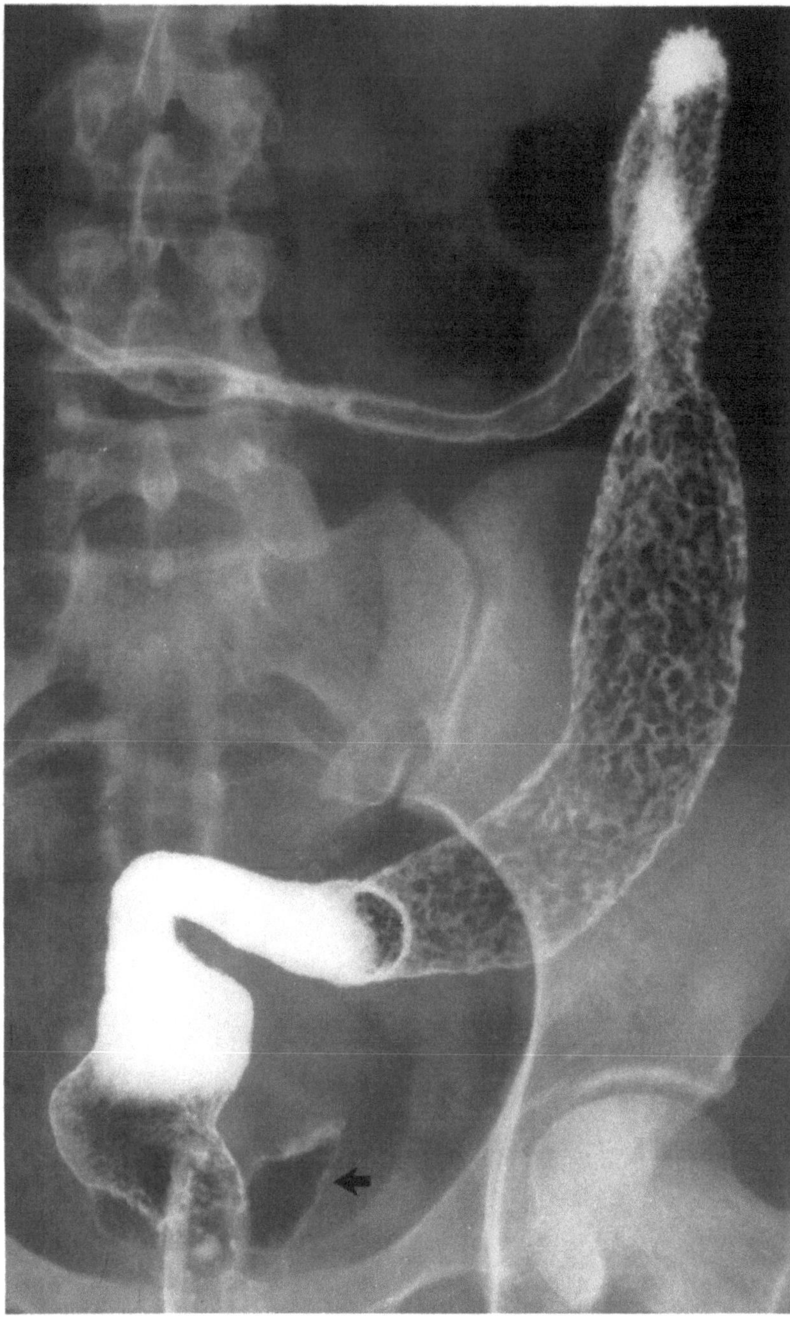

Fig. 6.11. Pseudopolypoid form of ulcerative colitis (patient in prone position): the numerous and adjoining pseudopolyps give the descending colon a cobblestoned appearance. Note the heterogeneous aspect and narrowed caliber of the rectal image and overall narrowing of the colon to the hepatic flexure. A blind anal fistula is also present *(arrow)*

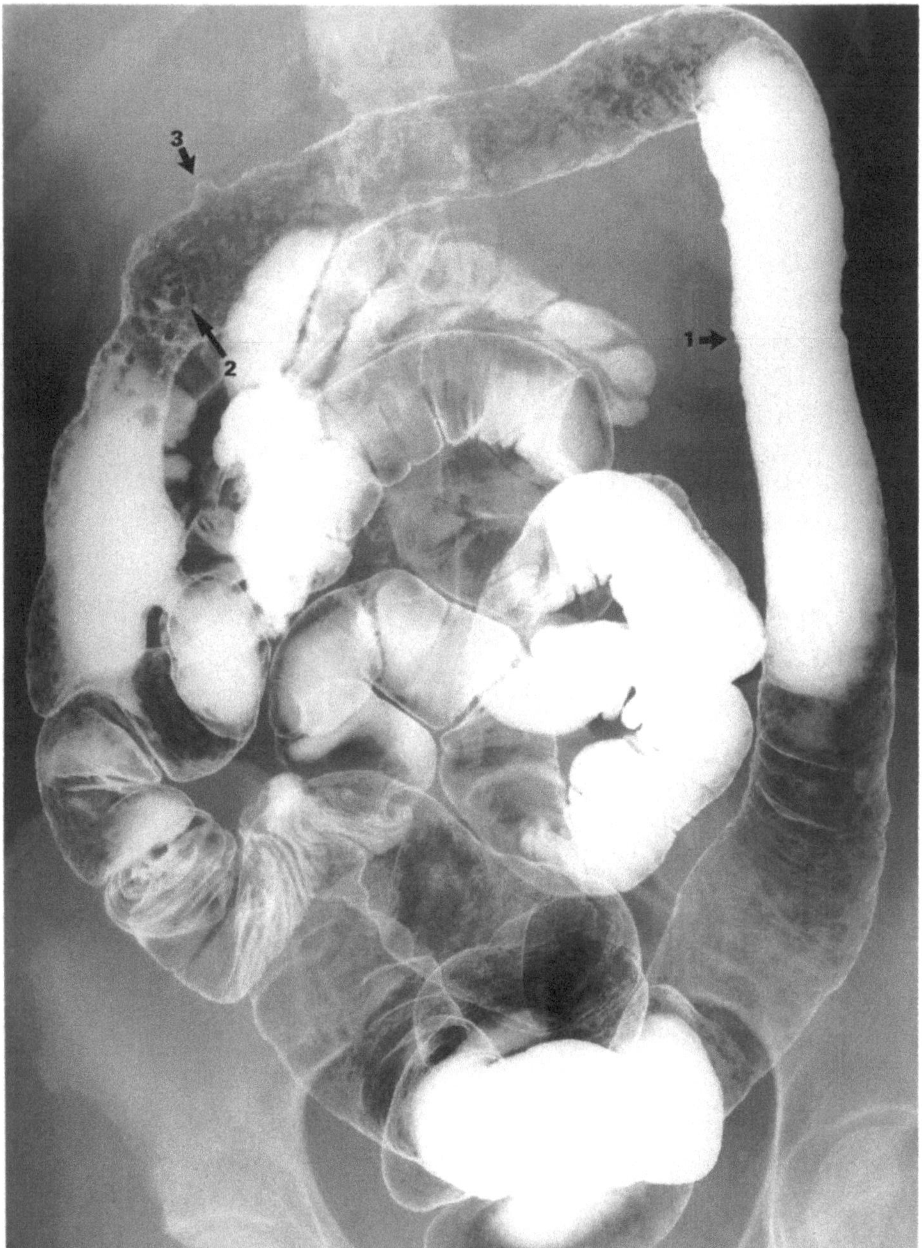

Fig. 6.12. Ulcerative colitis: ulceroproliferous stage in the right colon, ulcerative stage in the descending colon, and congestive stage in the sigmoid. The rectum and sigmoid have a reticular appearance. Ulcerations with caliber and haustral abnormalities are predominant in the descending colon and splenic flexure *(arrow 1)*. Pseudopolyps are seen in the hepatic flexure *(arrow 2)* with signs of retraction already present *(arrow 2)*. A pseudodiverticulum is present *(arrow 3)*

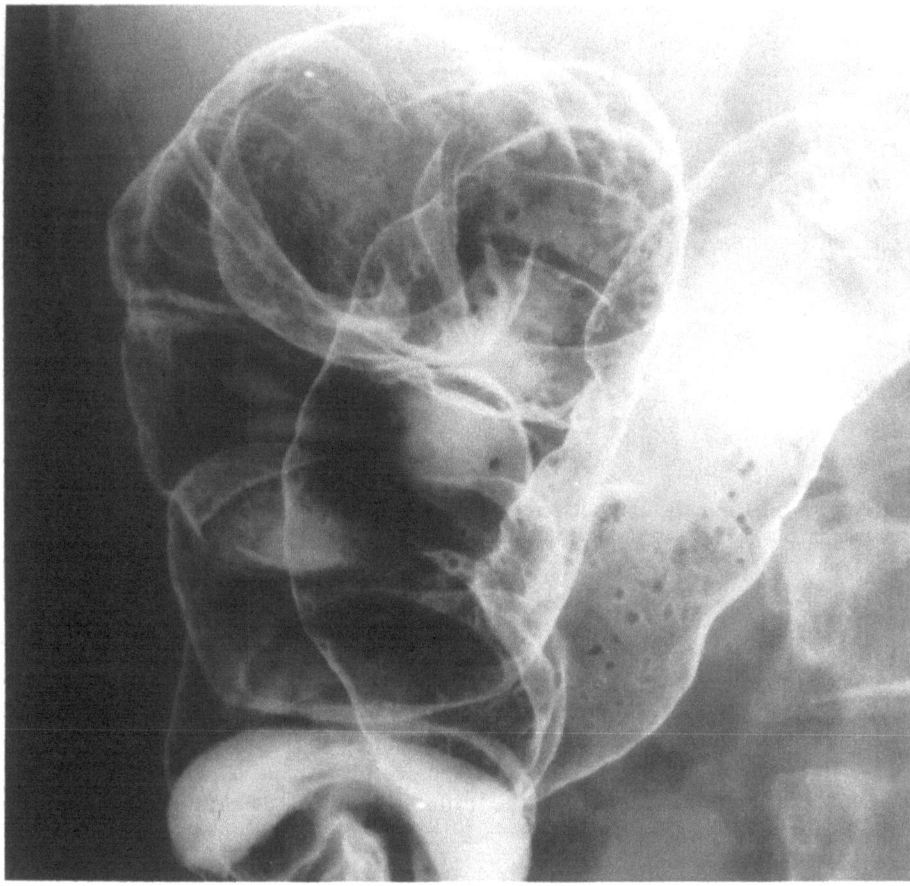

Fig. 6.13. Ulcerative colitis in remission. Small pseudopolyps spread throughout the hepatic flexure and transverse colon are clearly seen in the pool

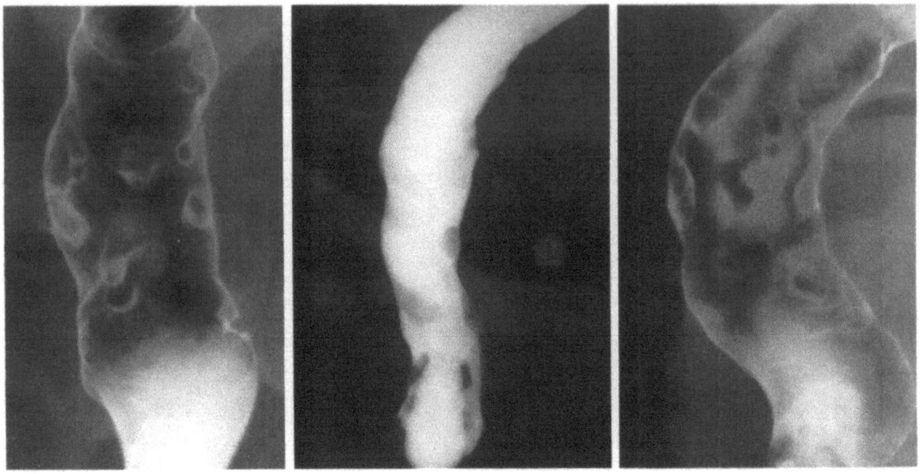

A, B, C

Fig. 6.14 A–C. Ulcerative colitis in remission. Pseudopolyps are seen in the rectal ampulla (some are digital polyps). Otherwise the mucosal appearance is normal

6.3 Differential Diagnosis

The granular aspect appears to be highly suggestive of but not specific to ulcerative colitis. Other characteristics include: the continuity, symmetry, regularity, and diffuseness of the lesions as well as the rectal involvement, proximal spread, and noninvolvement of the terminal ileum. These radiologic signs make it possible to diagnose 83% of cases [2].

References

1. Bret P, Piante M, Cuche C, Jeannot J (1976) Exploration radiologique en double contraste des recto colites hémorragiques. Ann Radiol 19: 292–302
2. Kelvin FM, Odoson TA, Rice RP, Garbutt JT, Bradenham B (1978) Double contrast barium enema in Crohn's disease and ulcerative colitis. Am J Roentgenol 131: 207–213
3. Lauffer I, Edward Mullens J, Hamilton J (1976) Correlation of endoscopy and double contrast radiography in the early stages of ulcerative and granulomatous colitis. Radiology 118: 1–5
4. Miller RE, Skucas J (1983) The radiological examination of the colon. Practical diagnosis. Nijhoff, Amsterdam pp 156–171
5. Potet F (1975) Anatomie pathologique de la recto colite hémorragique. Rev Prat 25: 15–26
6. Simpkins KC, Stevenson GW (1972) The modified Malmö double contrast barium enema in colitis: an assessment of its accuracy in reflecting sigmoïdoscopic findings. Brit J Radiol 45: 486–492
7. Welin S, Brahme F (1960) The double contrast method in ulcerative colitis. Acta Radiol 55: 257–271
8. Welin S, Welin G (1976) The double contrast examination of the colon. Experiences with the Welin modification. Thieme, Stuttgart

7 Crohn's Disease of the Colon

In Crohn's disease, as in ulcerative colitis, the anatomic/radiologic relationship is very close. Double contrast provides for an excellent study of the lesions even at an early stage. Radiologic/endoscopic correlations are excellent [2-7].

7.1 Pathology

Crohn's disease of the colon has certain pathologic features, which are reviewed here briefly.

7.1.1 Lesion Distribution

Lesion distribution is characterized by: (1) Its topography: involvement of the ileum in 50% of cases and noninvolvement of the rectum in 50% of cases. (2) Discontinuous involvement characterized by an alternation of normal and pathologic segments as well as the presence of small patches of normal tissue within generally diseased areas or pathologic "fragments" in otherwise normal segments [7]. This often gives the lesions an asymmetric character.

7.1.2 Stage of Disease

Lesions have variable appearances according to the stage of the disease.

Early Stage

1. According to Morson [6], aphthous ulcers are the first sign. Endoscopically, they are small (the size of a pinhead to several millimeters in diameter), generally rounded, and shallow with slightly raised borders [6-8]. They may be isolated or grouped together separated by intervals of normal mucosa.

2. Submucous edema due to lymphatic stasis is also considered to be an initial sign [6]. The mucosa may simply have an edematous or irregular appearance. According to Welin [9], submucous edema raises the mucosa forming transverse folds separated by fairly deep grooves.

Advanced Stages. Ulcerations enlarged in size, depth, or by the surrounding ring of edema are associated with or follow aphthous ulcers. Histologically, the presence of transmural fissures affecting the entire thickness of the wall is highly indicative. These fissures may give way to intramural abscesses (collar-button double contour) or internal or enterocutaneous fistulae. Macroscopically the ulcers have irregular contours and may be linear and narrow or serpiginous. Adjacent mucosa may be normal (this is highly characteristic) or raised by submucous edema. This juxtaposition of ulceration and mucous patches creates a cobblestoned appearance. Finger-like pseudopolyps may also develop but seem to occur less frequently than in ulcerative colitis. Definitive retractile lesions due to the parietal thickening and associated fibrosis develop fairly rapidly. These include: longitudinal shortening, often asymmetric single or multiple stenosis, and cobblestoned mucosa (even without ulceration) due to transmural fibrous scarring which irregularly retracts the mucosa [3].

Remissions. In early remissions, ulcers regress and the mucosa may return to normal. Subsequently, lesions as well as the cobblestoned aspect and pseudopolyps persist.

7.2 Correspondence of Radiologic Images to the Lesions

7.2.1 *Early Stage*

Aphthous ulcers and parietal edema are the most characteristic features.

7.2.1.1 Aphthous Ulcers

These appear on the walls as small opaque spots which are largely rounded and usually encircled by a radiolucent halo due to the surrounding edema. They form bull's-eye images (Figs. 7.1, 7.2). They are not always demonstrated along the border. They may appear as shallow, flat-bottomed or triangular addition images either projecting or in a filling defect (Figs. 7.2, 7.3).

In some cases the filling defect feature may be predominant, in which case we speak of round-bottomed, nodular marginal filling defects. Often these nodules are topped by an ulcer (Figs. 7.3, 7.4). It is difficult when confronted with multiple and adjoining images to identify the spaces separating nodules from ulcers surrounded by a ring of edema. The image density is variable. Ulcers may be single or multiple, grouped together or dispersed (Fig. 7.5). The adjoining mucosa may appear normal or irregular but rarely has the uniform granular appearance characteristic of ulcerative colitis. In more advanced stages, ulcers are especially found in a transition zone between normal and pathologic mucosa (Fig. 7.4) [12].

7.2.1.2 Barium Stagnation Between Edematous Mucous Folds

Barium stagnation between edematous mucous folds is considered (Welin [9]) an early sign of important diagnostic value. Transverse mucous folding occurs in the normal colon at rest but disappears with distension. In Crohn's disease submucous edema raises the mucosa creating these folds and their abnormal persistence. The resulting image is of straight, opaque transverse stripes several millimeters wide (as opposed to the arciform transverse lines formed by haustral contours) (Fig. 7.5). These opaque stripes are mainly associated with ulcerations. According to Welin [9], this is highly suggestive of Crohn's disease and is absent in ulcerative colitis.

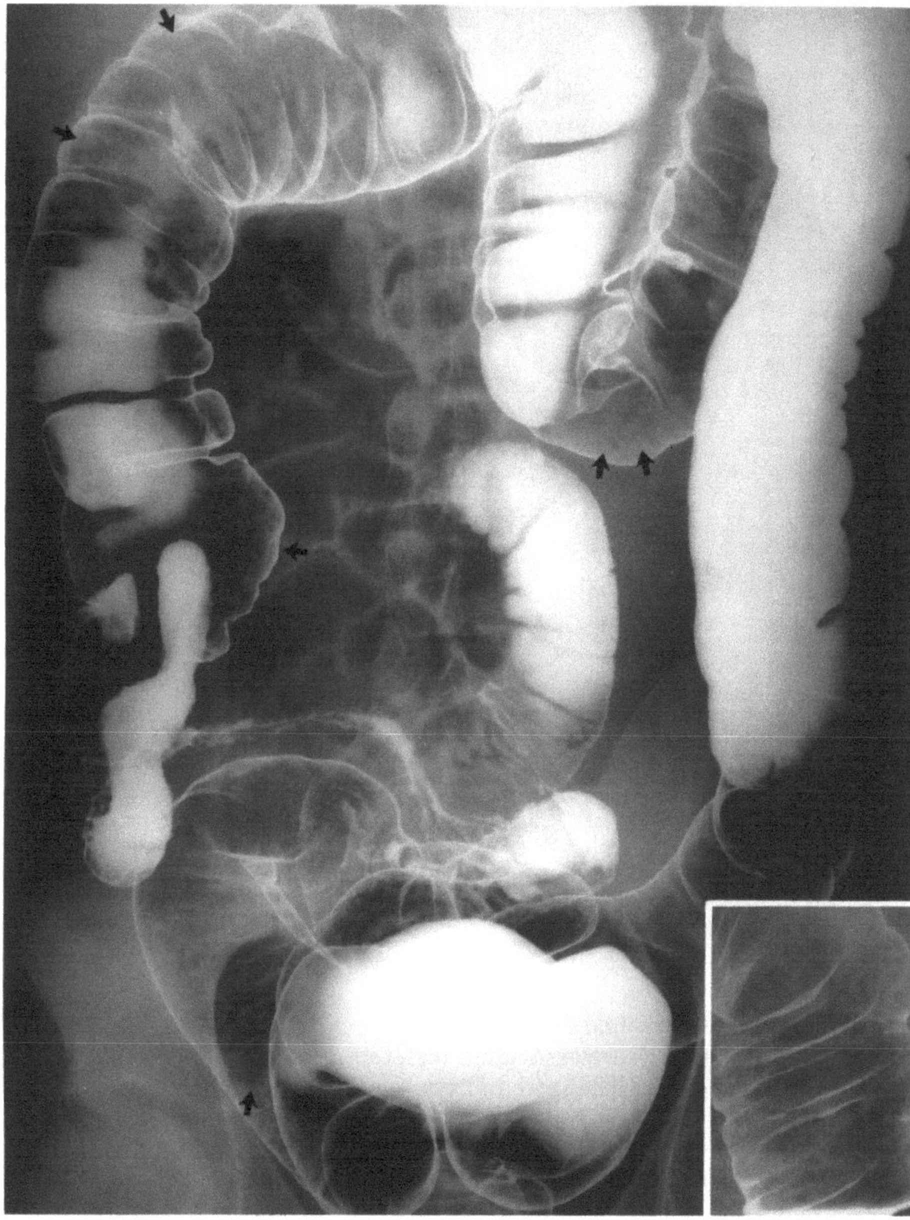

A B

Fig. 7.1. Ileocolonic Crohn's disease (courtesy of Dr. Recart, Pessac). **A** Note the typical involvement of the terminal ileum. Lesions of the colon are small aphthous ulcers represented by opaque spots surrounded by a ring of edema. **B** Descending segment of the hepatic flexure: ulcerations here are very distinct. The radiologic appearance is significantly different from that of physiologic microspiculation

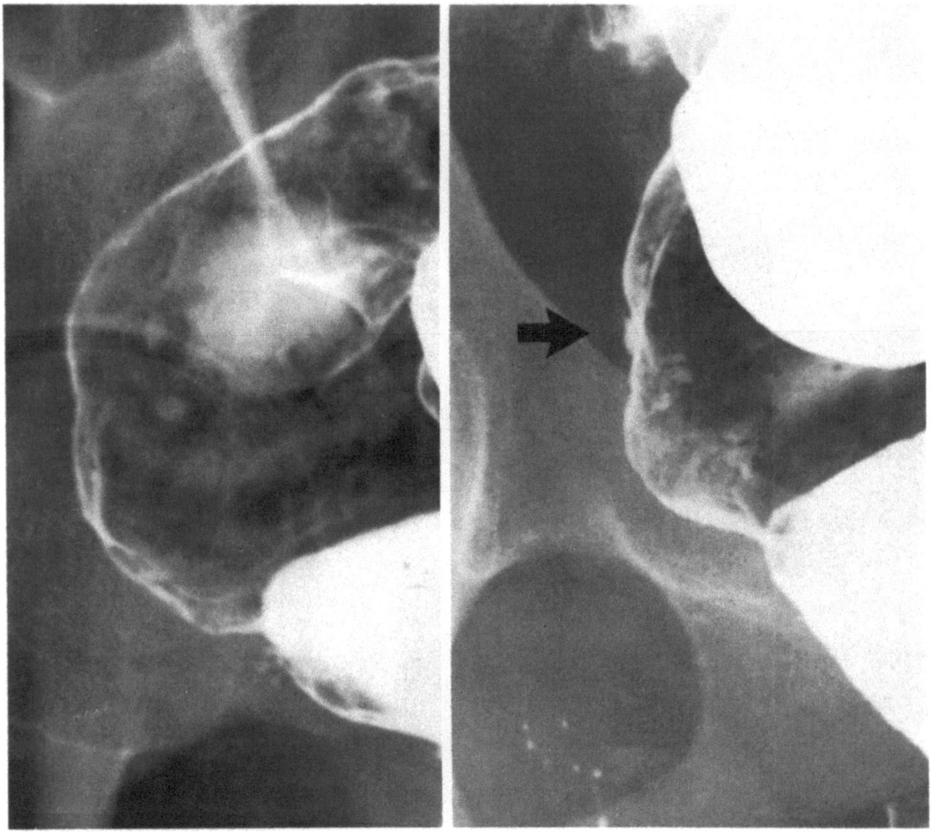

A B

Fig. 7.2. Ileocolonic Crohn's disease. Earliest features of rectal involvement. **A** Note the two opaque spots encircled by a radiolucent halo (bull's-eye image) corresponding to aphthous ulcers seen frontally. **B** In profile one of these ulcers is seen surrounded by a ring of edema *(arrow)*

7.2.1.3 Functional Abnormalities

Functional abnormalities are associated with these lesions. While nonspecific, they may be suggestive if localized and symmetric. They are concerned not so much with the spastic contraction of a diseased segment as with haustral modifications (reduction or localized loss with rigidity of one margin) or caliber abnormalities (overall symmetric or asymmetric narrowing of a segment). These defects seem to be relatively rare and discrete in the early stages and become more evident as the lesions develop.

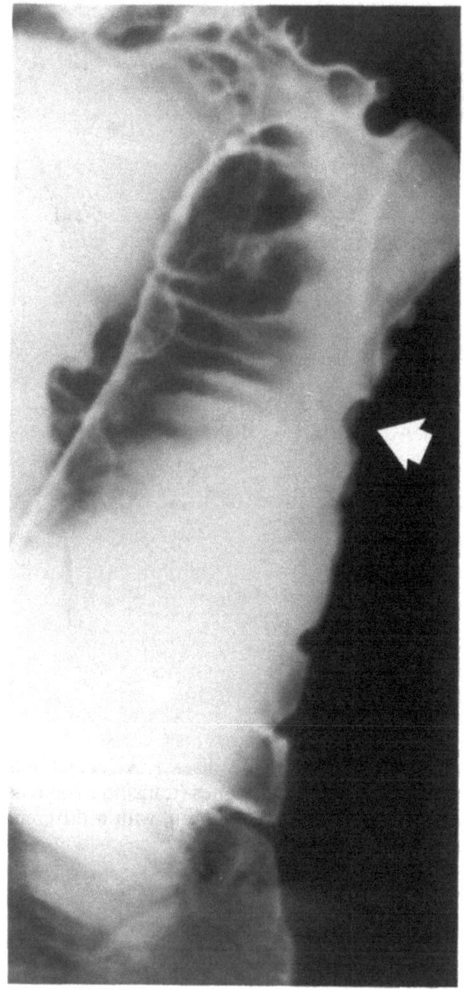

Fig. 7.3. Asymmetric involvement of the splenic flexure in ileocolonic Crohn's disease. Marginal filling defects *(arrow)* face "Welin's stripes". The half-tinted image at the bottom of the filling defect corresponds to an ulcer. These filling defects are localized on a patch of the colonic segment in question

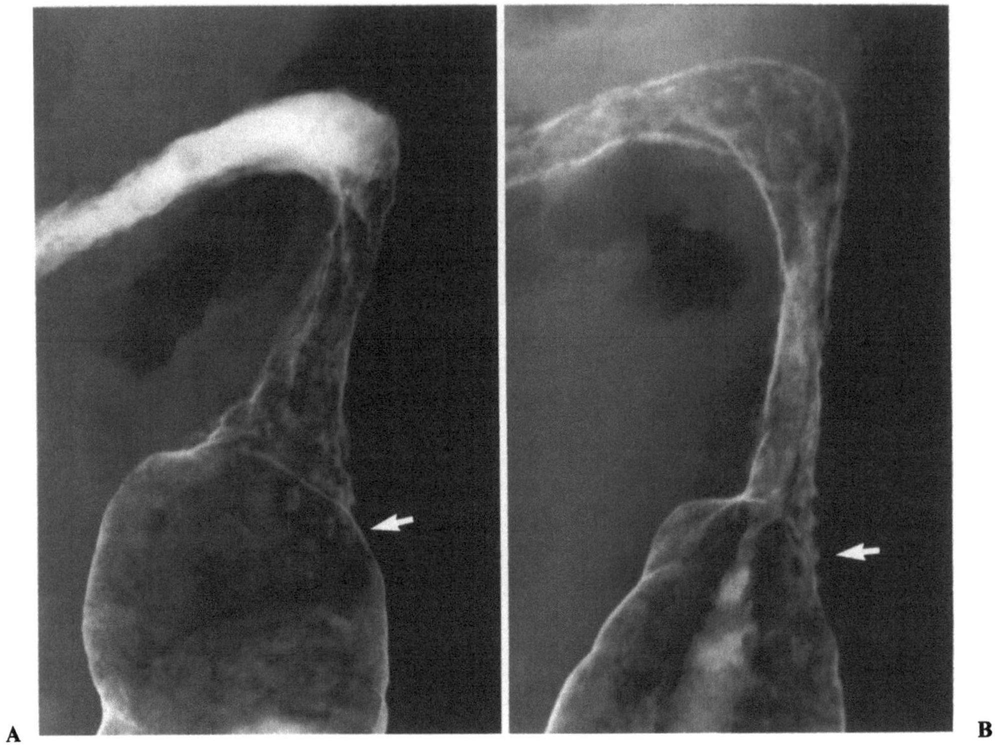

Fig. 7.4. Colonic Crohn's disease. **A** Several bull's-eye images grouped together at the junction of normal and pathologic zones (transition zone) correspond to aphthous ulcers *(arrow)*. **B** These images are seen along the margin, with a different incident angle, as addition images separated by small filling defects

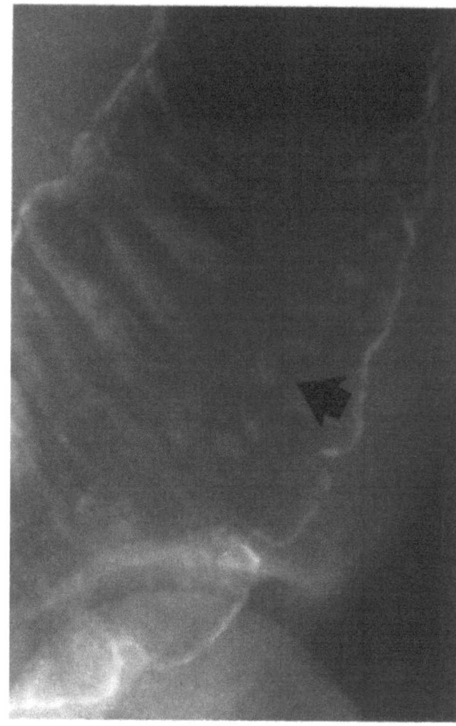

Fig. 7.5. Colonic Crohn's disease with sigmoid involvement. Dispersed aphthous ulcers with "Welin's stripes"

7.2.2 Advanced Stages

Advanced stages may sometimes be reached quite rapidly and lesions at different stages may coexist.(Figs. 7.6, 7.7).

1. Ulcers are more numerous and deeper: they are represented frontally as larger sized opaque spots with irregular contours arranged longitudinally or serpiginously. In profile they are clearly visualized and have diverse appearances (Fig. 7.6):

a) Triangular top: rose-bush thorn (Fig. 7.8), horn, or raspberry-bush thorn

b) Flat-bottomed (Fig. 7.9), notched, collar-button or double contour when intramural detachments occur (Fig. 7.10)

c) Deep fissures may also be seen (Fig. 7.11)

Cobblestoned mucosa may be present and is due to the juxtaposition of two elements: filling defects or images circled by barium (mucous remnants or inflammatory pseudopolyps) giving the margins a sawtooth or jagged-edged appearance and intersecting opaque lines separating these images due to the stagnation of barium in the ulcerations or transverse grooves. The resulting cobblestoned mucosa varies in appearance depending on the predominant feature: large ulcerations (Fig. 7.12), nodular images (Fig. 7.13), or transverse grooves (Fig. 7.14).

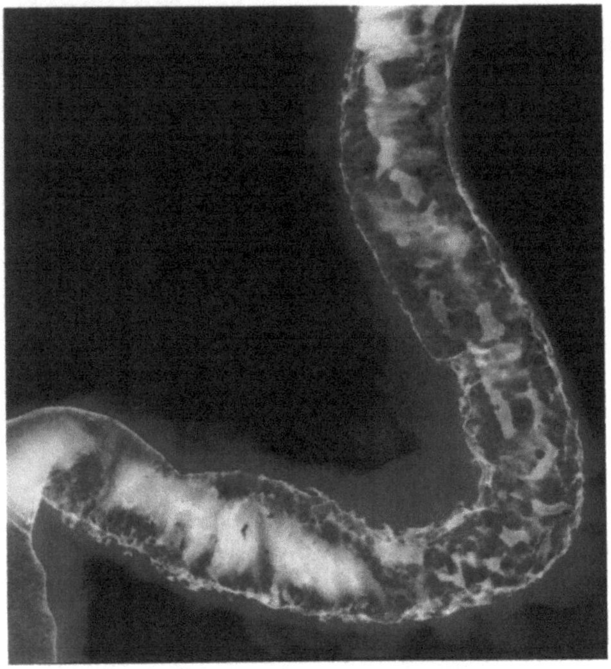

A

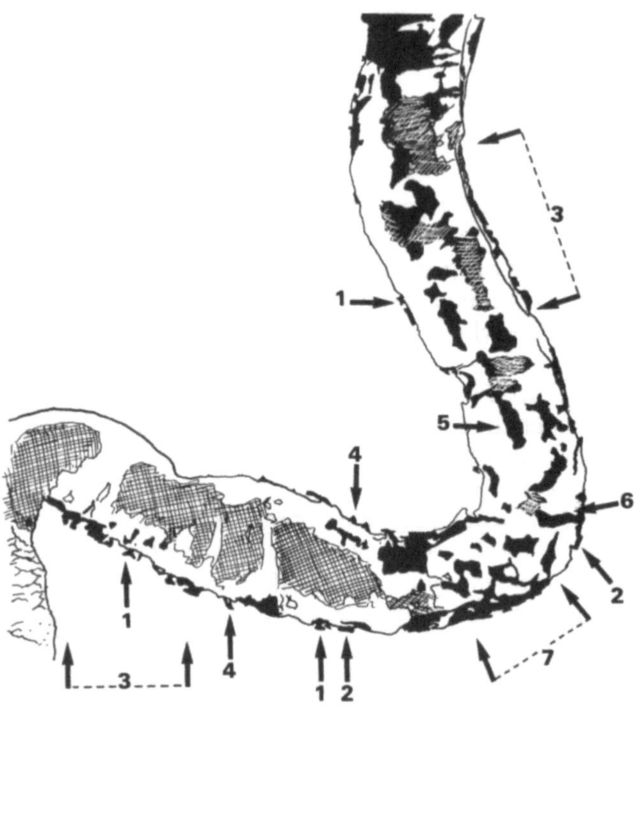

B

Fig. 7.6 A, B. Ileocolonic Crohn's disease. Radiograph of the rectosigmoid and left colon. Different types of ulcers can be seen:
1. As addition images along the margins: **1** collar-button (T-shape), **2** notched, **3** double contour, and **4** thorn
2. In the intermarginal aspect, as spots with irregular contours: **5** arranged longitudinally, **6** transversally, and **7** serpiginously

2. Caliber abnormalities at this stage most often result from major parietal hypertrophy and irreversible fibrous lesions. In the most highly diseased segments the narrowed caliber accentuates the difference between these and normal areas. Major longitudinal retraction may occur in widespread forms (Fig. 7.11). Single or multiple stenosis, usually asymmetric but sometimes concentric, may develop.

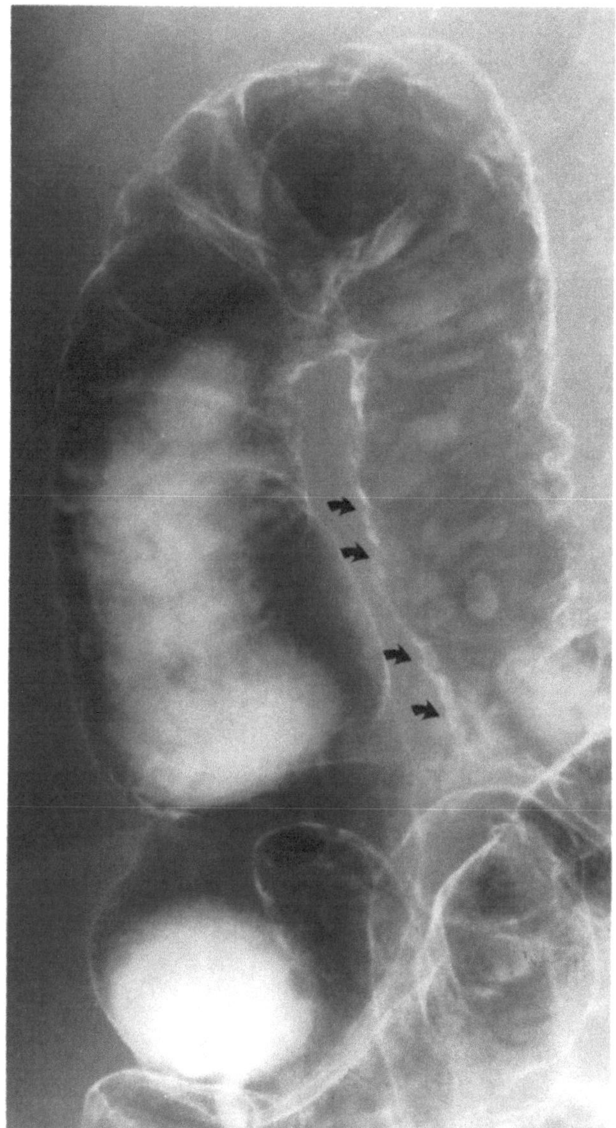

Fig. 7.7. Crohn's disease of the right colon. Deep ulcers are seen frontally (bull's-eye) and in profile *(arrows)*. The overall caliber is narrowed with a loss of haustration

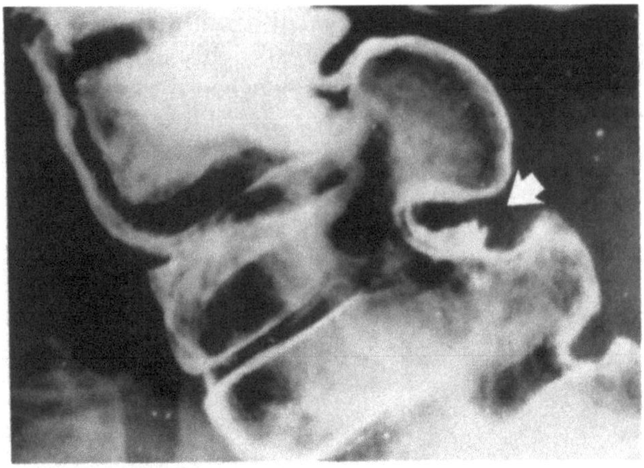

Fig. 7.8. Colonic Crohn's disease: deep, isolated "rose-bush thorn" ulcer *(arrow)*

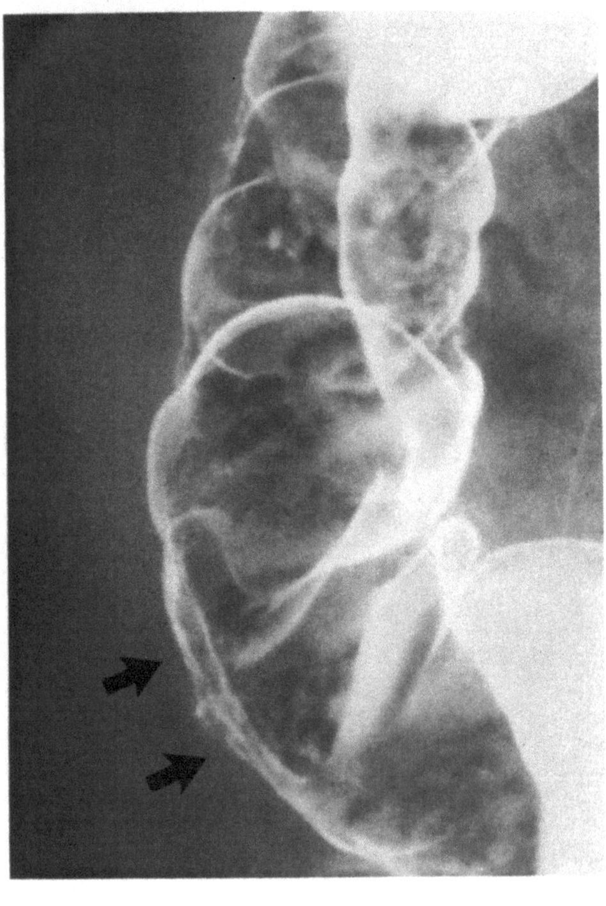

Fig. 7.9. Colonic Crohn's disease: longitudinal ulcer with raised margins. The base appears by the tangent effect as a line which doubles the colonic margin

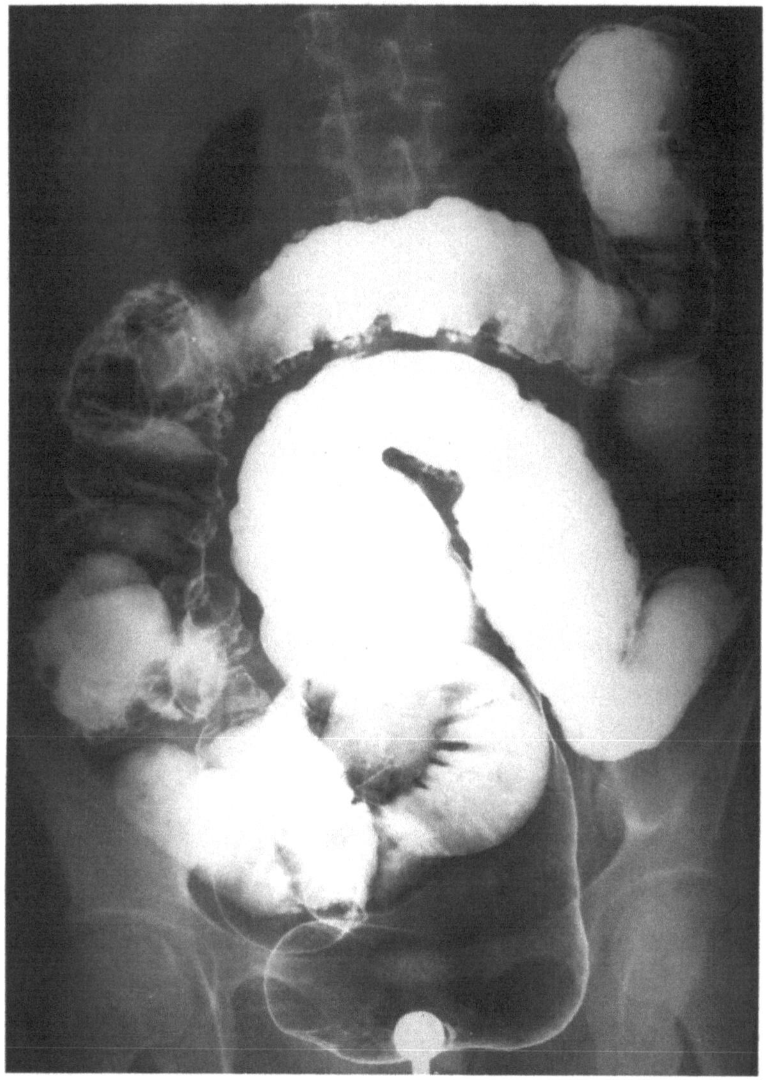

Fig. 7.10. Ileocolonic Crohn's disease: discontinuous lesions. The mucosa of the rectum and a short segment of the descending colon appear normal. Otherwise, the involvement is evident, notably by intramural abscesses with a double contour appearance on the transverse colon and part of the sigmoid. Note the asymmetric involvement of the margins of the transverse and sigmoid colon

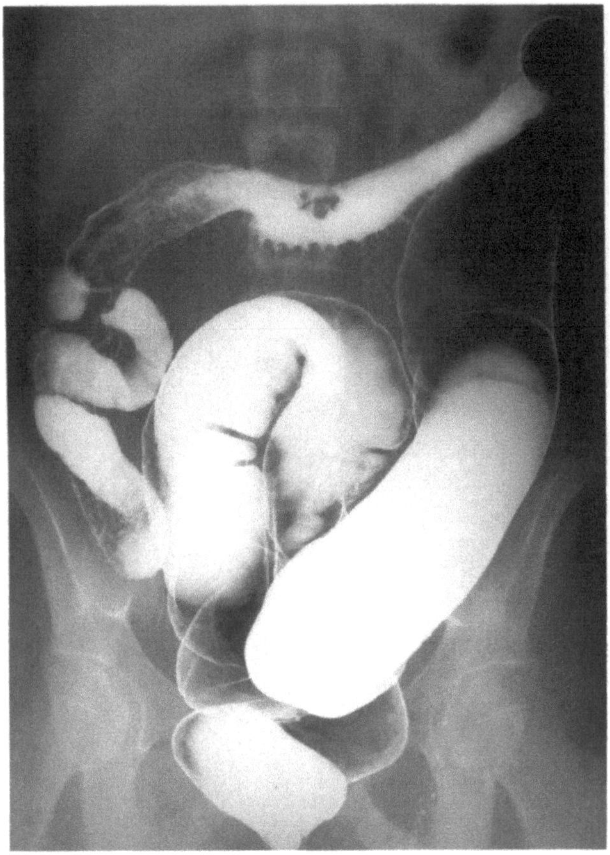

Fig. 7.11. Ileocolonic Crohn's disease. Major retraction of the entire right and transverse colons. Deep ulcerations with irregular contours on the inferior margin of the transverse colon. The radiograph also shows ulcerations on the cecal walls, pseudopolypoid (filling defect) images in the transverse colon, involvement of the terminal ileum, and a normal rectum

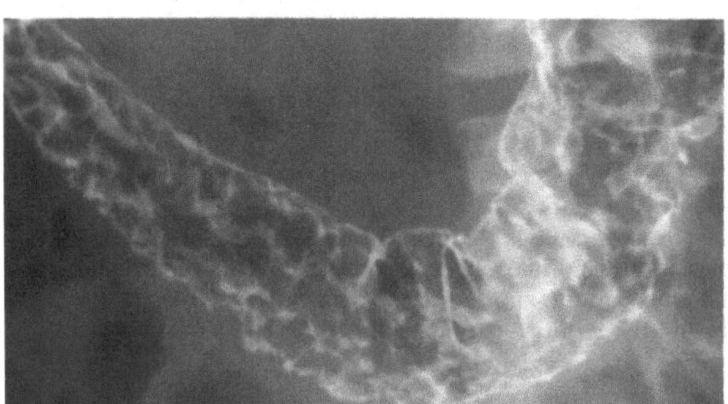

Fig. 7.12. Serpiginous ulcerations of the transverse colon in ileocolonic Crohn's disease. Cobblestoned appearance

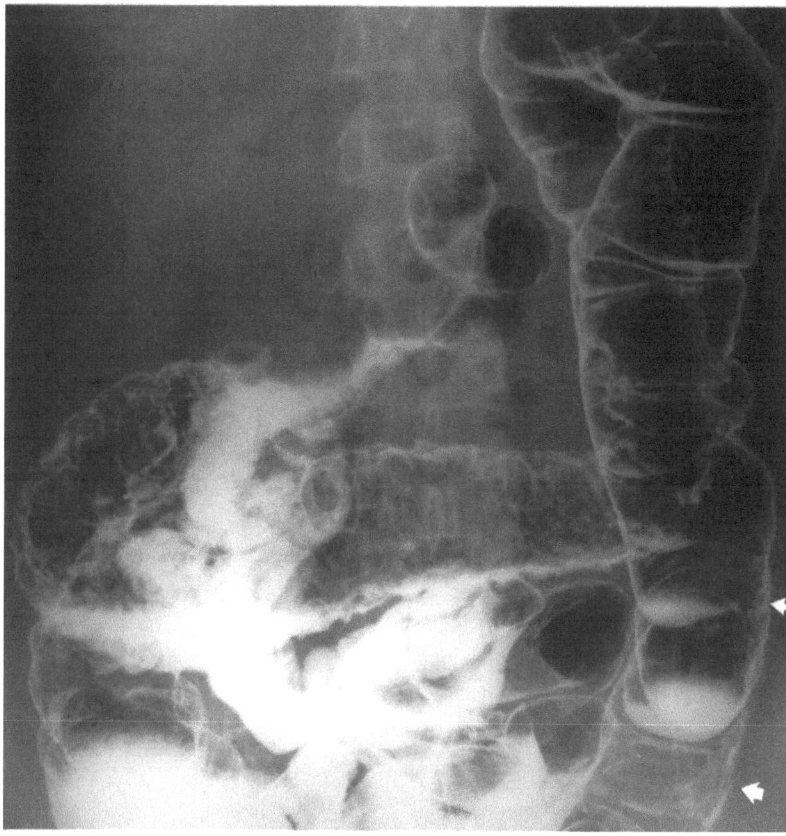

Fig. 7.13. Colonic Crohn's disease. Cobblestoned appearance of the transverse colon and hepatic flexure. The descending segment of the splenic flexure is normal (discontinuous involvement). Ulcerations are present in the descending colon *(arrows)*

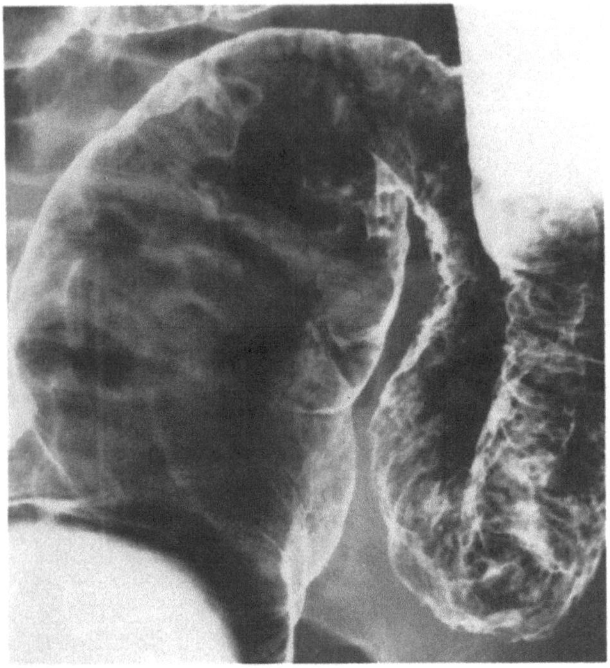

Fig. 7.14. Another cobblestoned image. Ulcerations, nodular images, and transverse grooves can be seen

7.2.3 Remissions

At an early stage, even following acute attacks, the colon may resume an almost normal appearance (Figs. 7.15, 7.16). The presence of pseudopolyps may indicate previous acute attacks (Fig. 7.17). In more advanced forms, cobblestoned scarring persists. Its contours, however, are better delimited and more distinct than during acute attacks. Stenosis and retractions are permanent. Sacculations may form due to intramural fibrous scarring (Fig. 7.18). These are highly suggestive of Crohn's disease since they demonstrate its discontinuous character. Sacculations correspond to areas of normal expansion surrounded by retracted fibrous zones.

7.2.4 Diagnostic Value of Radiologic Signs

The radiologic appearance of certain lesions (aphthous ulcers) and the arrangement or distribution of lesions in the colon (discontinuity, fragmented as opposed to circumferential involvement, topography) have an important diagnostic value.

7.2.4.1 Aphthous Ulcers

While not specific the presence of aphthous ulcers is highly characteristic. Identical images have been observed in Behçet's syndrome, Yersinia enterocolitis, amebic colitis, and leukopenia [4].

7.2.4.2 Discontinuous Nature

The discontinuous nature as seen in an alternation of segments showing ulcerations, haustral modifications, and reduced caliber with segments showing normal expansibility, haustrations, and mucosa (Figs. 7.13, 7.18–7.20).

7.2.4.3 Patched Versus Circumferential Character

The patched versus circumferential character of the disease can be seen in segments which are generally normal as well as which are those mainly pathologic. A pathologic "patch" in a generally normal segment (Figs. 7.2, 7.3, 7.8) is represented by several ulcers, a few marginal filling defects, or the rigidity of a retracted margin. The other margin retains its normal expansibility, giving the affected segment an asymmetric appearance. Subsequently, continued retraction may cause sacculation of the colonic wall. On the other hand, patches of less affected or even normal mucosa may be found in colonic segments of severe disease and narrowed caliber (Fig. 7.19).

7.2.4.4 Characteristic Topography of the Lesions

The rectum is frequently unaffected in Crohn's disease. This is clearly shown by double contrast and is an important factor. Terminal ileal reflux is frequent and should be carefully studied (Fig. 7.20). Involvement here is an important element for differential diagnosis especially in cases of diffuse colonic involvement. The predominance of lesions in the right colon is classic. It should be not-

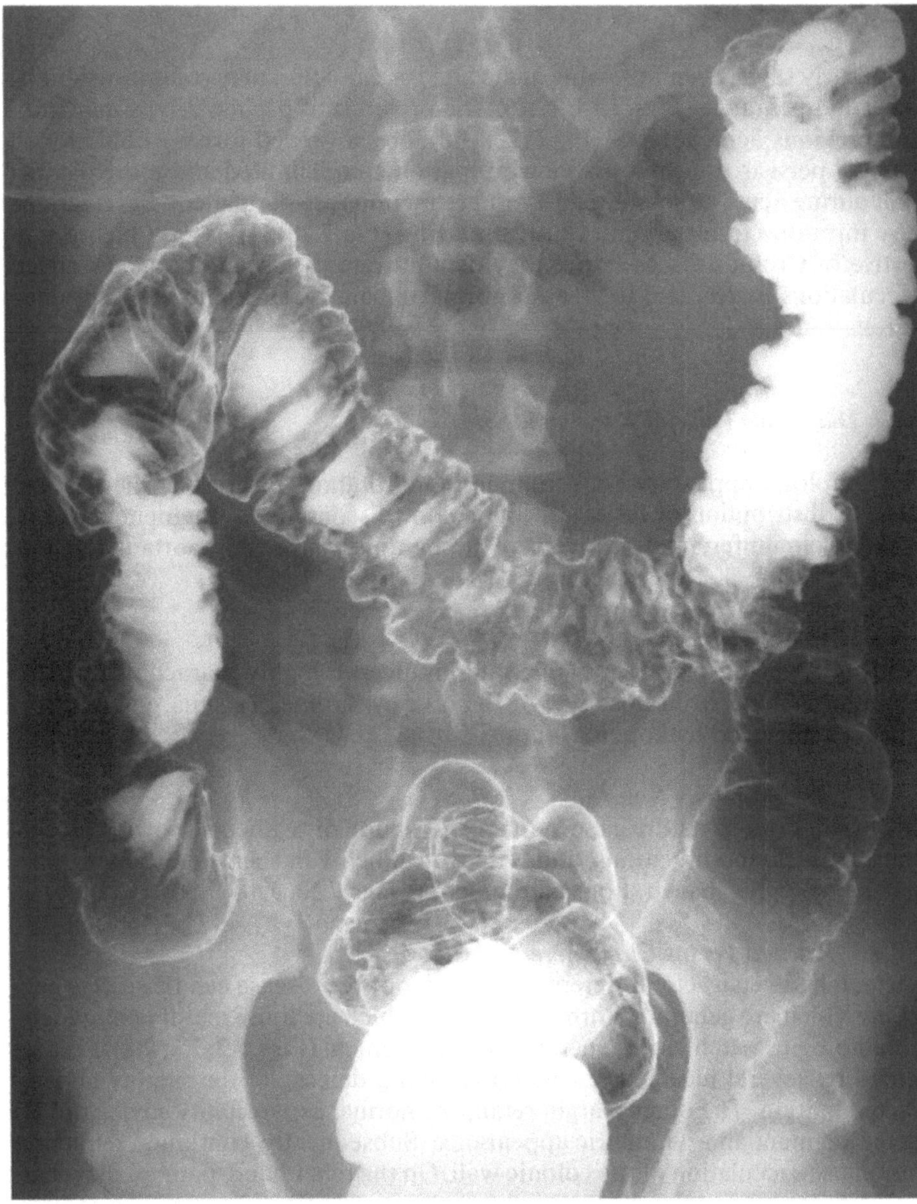

Fig. 7.15. Ileocolonic Crohn's disease. First examination 2 months after the initial symptoms. Different stages of lesions can be seen: the double contrast image of the proximal sigmoid and iliac colon is heterogeneous due to numerous small superficial ulcerations (similar to ulcerative colitis). In the splenic flexure, transverse colon and hepatic flexure, haustra are irregular, asymmetric, and sometimes inversed; ulcerations are found on the walls and some are encircled by a radiolucent halo and have irregular contours; marginal ulcerations have variable forms. Lesions are larger in the ascending colon. The caliber is narrowed. Folds are highly edematous and ulcerations are visible. This caliber reduction is not fixed (Fig. 7.16). A spasmodic factor intervenes

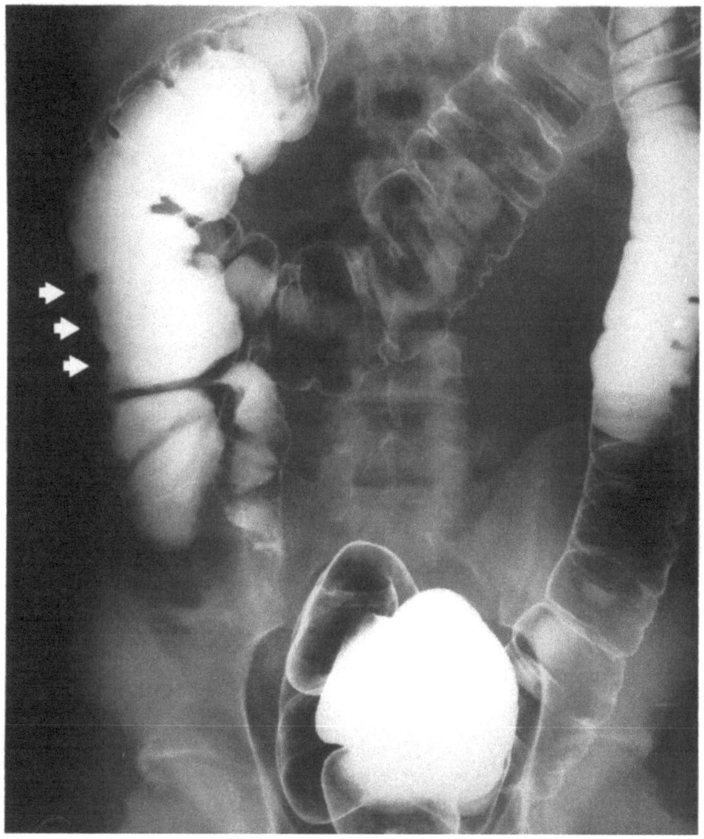

Fig. 7.16. Ileocolonic Crohn's disease (same patient as in Fig. 7.15). During remission, after the initial acute attack, the colon resumed a normal appearance except in the cecum and ascending colon, where the most severe lesions developed. A certain rigidity and lacunar appearance of the lateral margin persist *(arrows)*

ed, however, that in the absence of any cecal localization, ileal involvement may cause extrinsic modifications of the cecum such as: compression and incurvation of its medial aspect.

7.2.5 Complications

Other than stenosis (Fig. 7.20) complications include internal or enterocutaneous fistulae. Malignant change is less frequent than in ulcerative colitis but is possible. Toxic megacolon is a contraindication for all barium enemas.

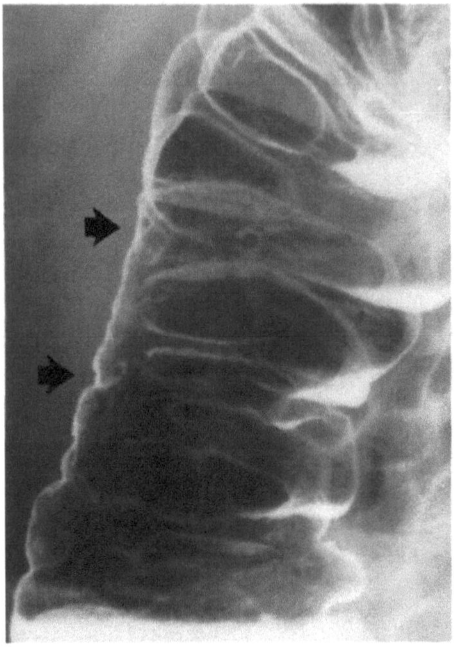

Fig. 7.17. Same patient as in Figs. 7.15 and 7.16. Localized films showing pseudopolyps and confirm the rigidity of the lateral margin

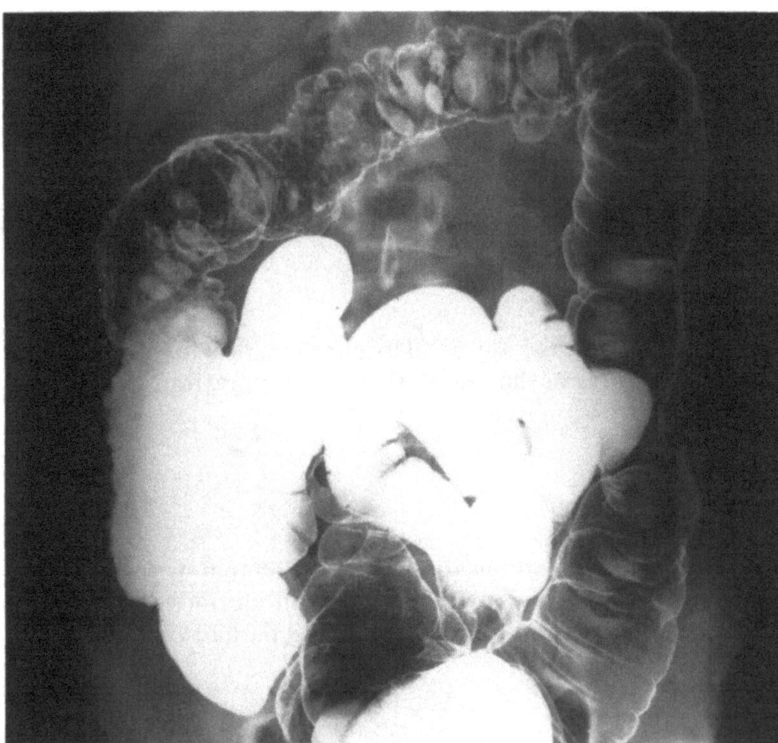

Fig. 7.18

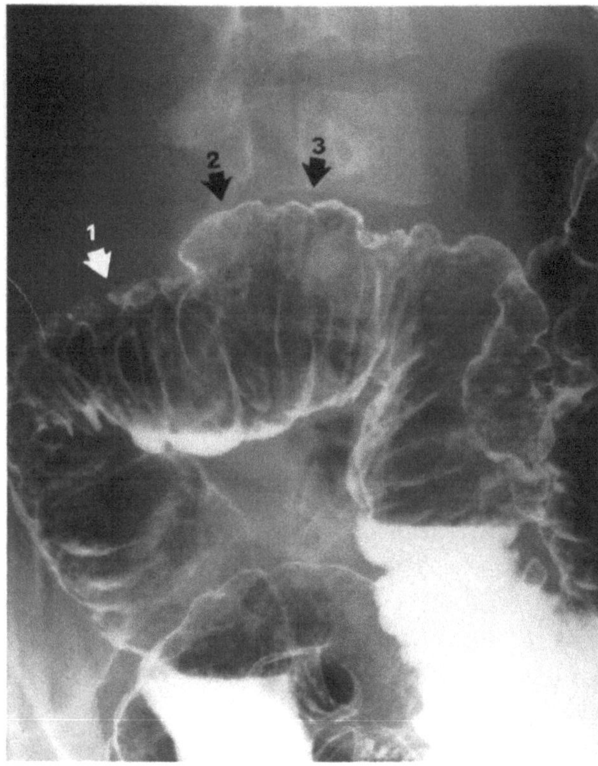

Fig. 7.19. Colonic Crohn's disease: asymmetric nature of the involvement: adjacent to a highly pathologic zone **(1)** is a patch of apparently normal mucosa **(2)**. Ulcerations can be seen several centimeters away **(3)**

◁ **Fig. 7.18.** Colonic Crohn's disease: discontinuous lesions and pseudodiverticular appearance in the transverse colon. (Courtesy of Pr Benaceraff, Paris)

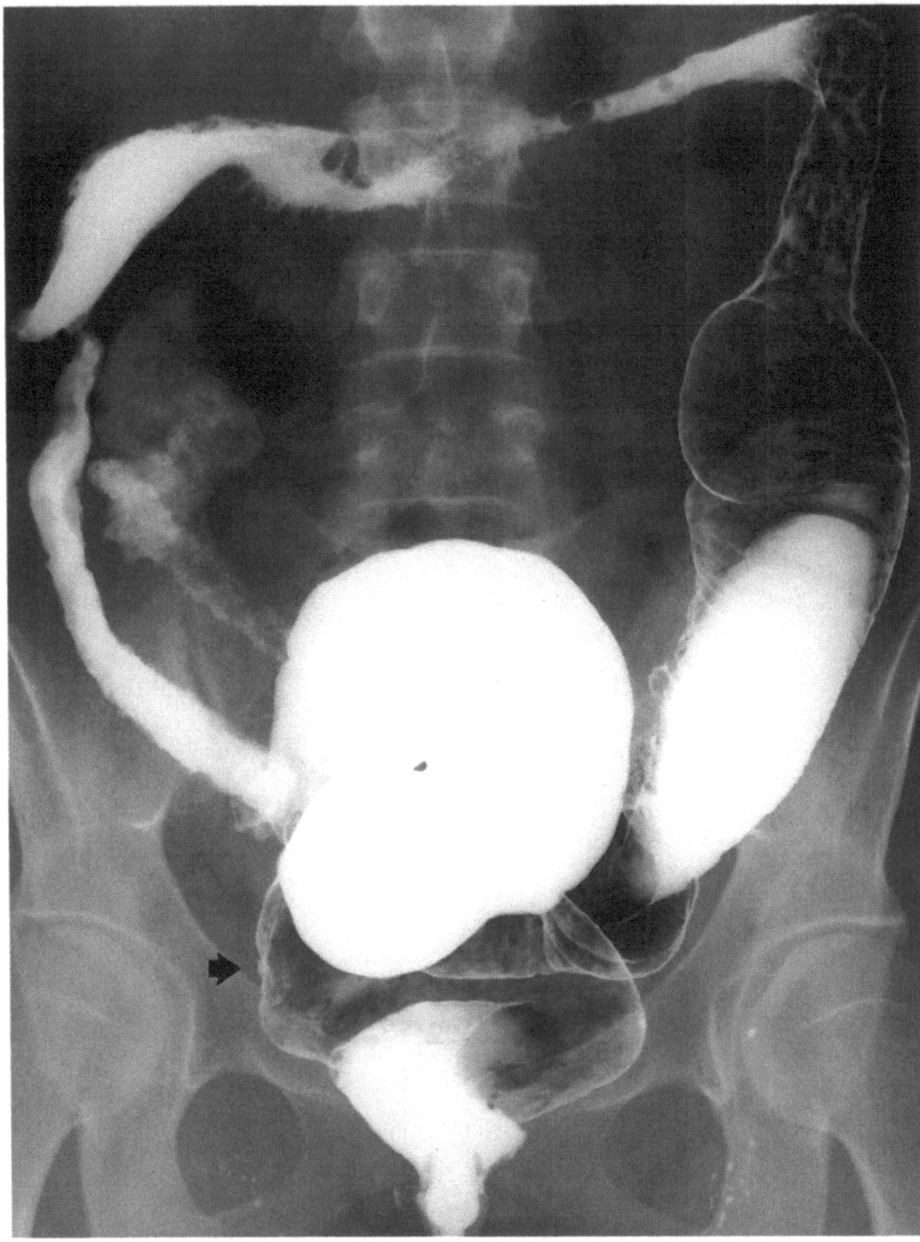

Fig. 7.20. Advanced ileocolonic Crohn's disease: long and rigid asymmetric stenosis. Several ulcerations indicate rectal involvement *(arrow)*. Involvement of the splenic flexure

7.3 Conclusion

Double contrast provides for a satisfactory examination of patients with Crohn's disease. Early lesions as well as the discontinuous nature of the disease are clearly shown. Diagnosis by double contrast is possible in 94%-98% of cases [1-11].

References

1. Kelvin FM, Oddson TA, Rice RP, Garbutt JT, Bradenham BP (1978) Double contrast barium enema in Crohn's disease and ulcerative colitis. Am J Roentgenol 131: 207-213
2. Laufer I, Mullens JE, Hamilton J (1976) Correlation of endoscopy and double contrast radiography in the early stages of ulcerative and granulomatous colitis. Radiology 118: 1-5
3. Marshak RH (1975) Granulomatous disease of the intestinal tract. Radiology 114: 3-22
4. Max RJ, Kelvin F (1980) Non specificity of discrete colonic ulceration on double contrast enema study. Am J Roentgenol 134: 1265-1267
5. Miller RE, Skucas J (1983) The radiological examination of the colon. Nijhoff, Amsterdam pp 135-153
6. Morson BC, Dawson IMP (1979) Gastrointestinal pathology, 2nd edn. Blackwell, Oxford pp 293-310
7. Simpkins KC (1976) The barium enema in Crohn's colitis. In: The management of Crohn's disease. Proceedings of the workshop on Crohn's disease. Leyden, oct 1975. Excerpta Medica, Amsterdam-Oxford, pp 62-67
8. Vantrappen G (1976) A prospective study of colonoscopy in Crohn's disease. In: The management of Crohn's disease. Proceedings of the workshop on Crohn's disease. Excerpta Medica, Amsterdam-Oxford, pp 79-83
9. Welin S, Welin G (1973) A pathognomonic roentgenologic sign of regional ileitis (Crohn's disease). Dis Col Rect 16: 473-478
10. Welin S, Welin G (1976) The double contrast examination of the colon. Experiences with the Welin modification. Thieme, Stuttgart
11. Williams HJ, Stephens DH, Carlson HC (1981) Double contrast radiography: colonic inflammatory disease. AJR 137: 315-322
12. Young A (1968) Radiologie de la maladie inflammatoire du côlon. Actual hepato-gastro-enterol Masson Paris 4: 217-231

8 Colonic Diverticulosis

Diverticulosis is the most frequent colonic disease today in the Western industrial nations. The sigmoid colon is the segment most frequently affected. The radiologic image generally demonstrates two features: diverticular pouches and distortion of the colonic lumen. Discovery of diverticula confirm the diagnosis. Distortion of the sigmoid lumen, which frequently accompanies diverticular formation, was for a long time and is still sometimes misinterpreted as a sign of diverticulitis.

8.1 Physiopathogenic Review

The pathogenicity of diverticulosis is still poorly understood. According to the oldest theory [1-11], increased intraluminal pressure in small localized segments pushes the mucosa through weak points in the colonic wall where vessels penetrate the circular muscle. Recently Taylor [13] demonstrated, a myoelectric slow-wave pattern at an abnormal frequency of 12 cpm, which disappeared following the ingestion of bran. Whatever the exact mechanism, the muscular abnormalities characteristic of the disease would be due to prolonged hyperactivity itself secondary to a low-fiber diet. Some diverticula (isolated diverticula, diverticula in the absence of muscular defects, more frequent in the right colon) may be due to a pathogenic mechanism different from that of common sigmoid diverticulosis.

8.2 Pathology Review

Three points should be considered: (1) the normal structure of the colonic muscular coat and the development of diverticula, (2) defects in the muscular coat which are usually present in this disease, and (3) the principal patterns of diverticular inflammation.

8.2.1 Development and Site of Diverticula

The muscular coat of the colon contains two layers: an external longitudinal layer and an internal circular layer. The longitudinal muscle is thin and is reinforced by three teniae. They arise from the base of the appendix and run the en-

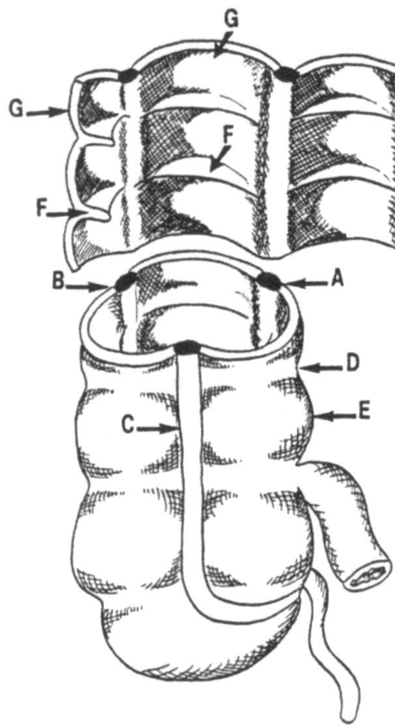

Fig. 8.1. Normal position of colonic teniae in the right colon. Here, as in the descending colon, the mesenteric tenia is medial **(A)** and the antimesenteric teniae are lateral **(B)** and anterior **(C)**. The division of the colonic circumference into three intertenial ridges is obvious. They include the antimesenteric ridge (between **B** and **C**) and two mesenteric ridges (between **A** and **C**, between **A** and **B**). Transverse grooves visible from the exterior **(D)** correspond to the normal valves or haustral clefts **(F)** visible from within. They delimit bulges **(E)** corresponding to the haustra (haustral cul-de-sacs) **(G)**

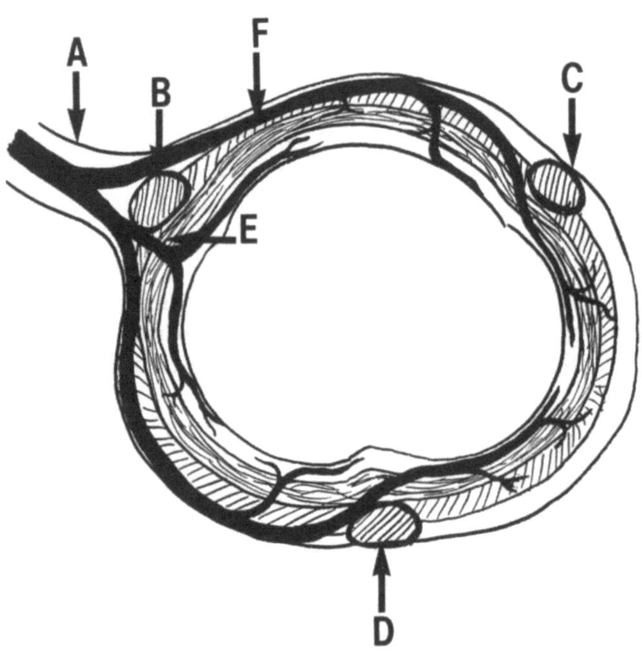

Fig. 8.2. Disposition of colonic vascularization. Penetration points of the muscular coat are adjacent to the mesenteric tenia **(B)** and on the mesocolic side of the antimesenteric teniae **(C and D)** (Meyers) [7]. The mesocolon **(A)**, mesenteric tenia **(B)**, antimesenteric teniae **(C, D)**, and short vasa recta **(E)** penetrate the muscular coat adjacent to the mesenteric tenia. **F**, long vasa recta

tire length of the colon. The mesenteric tenia corresponds to the mesocolon or at least to those segments joined to the paracolic vascular arch. The two antimesenteric teniae are at a distance. These three bands delimit three intertenial ridges (two mesenteric and one antimesenteric; Fig. 8.1).

At the sigmoid level, the two antimesenteric teniae draw together and become indistinguishable at the rectum [15]. The circular muscle is formed of muscular fibers and bundles arranged in small packets fastened to the tenia. It is between these bundles that the mucosa protrudes [15].

A diverticulum is a mucosal hernia through the circular muscle. Its wall is composed of the mucosa and submucous coat and is covered by the longitudinal muscle layer, serosa, and peritoneal fat. Actually, the thin longitudinal muscular layer is discontinuous and tears when a diverticulum reaches a certain size. It squeezes the diverticular neck, which may become occluded during contractions [14].

Macroscopically the diverticulum first forms a "herniated point" which is a small conical or cup-shaped expansion. Subsequently, a spherical pouch several millimeters to several centimeters in diameter develops. It is attached to the wall by a narrow zone, the neck. The diverticular orifice may become obstructed by fecal residue or during a contraction.

Site. The usual site of diverticula corresponds to areas of connective tissue where the vasa recta penetrate the muscular coat (Fig. 8.2). The arrangement of these weak spots and their relationship to the vessels has been the subject of numerous studies. According to Meyers [7], colonic vessels arise from the paracolic arch and approach the colon along the mesenteric tenia. They include the short vasa recta and long vasa recta. The former penetrate the muscular coat near the mesenteric tenia and the latter near the antimesenteric teniae after coursing through the subserosa (Fig. 8.2).

Vascular penetration points, then, are distributed on each side of the mesenteric tenia and the mesocolic side of the antimesenteric teniae. Diverticula are equally arranged in four rows on the mesenteric intertenial ridges (Fig. 8.3). It is this four-row arrangement that should be kept in mind; however, this description is incomplete. Though rare, diverticula may develop in the antimesenteric intertenial ridge outside the vascular territory. These diverticula which remain small have no clinical significance [8, 9, 14].

Diverticular Distribution in the Colon. Predominance in the sigmoid colon is clear (85% according to Bertrand [2]). Diverticula may appear anywhere in the colon (diffuse forms, 10%) but almost never in the rectum. Bertrand notes an exclusive radiologic localization of the disease in the right colon in 40% of cases. During autopsies, however, Hughes [6] has been unable to confirm these exclusive right forms.

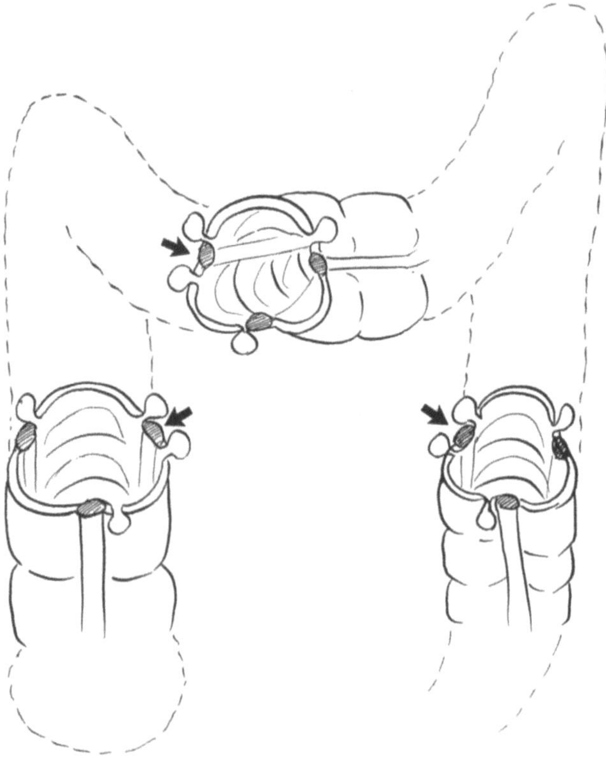

Fig. 8.3. Arrangement of diverticula in the colon: the position of the mesenteric tenia *(arrow)* varies according to the segment in question. Diverticula are found essentially on either side of the mesenteric tenia and the mesocolic side of the antimesenteric teniae

A

B

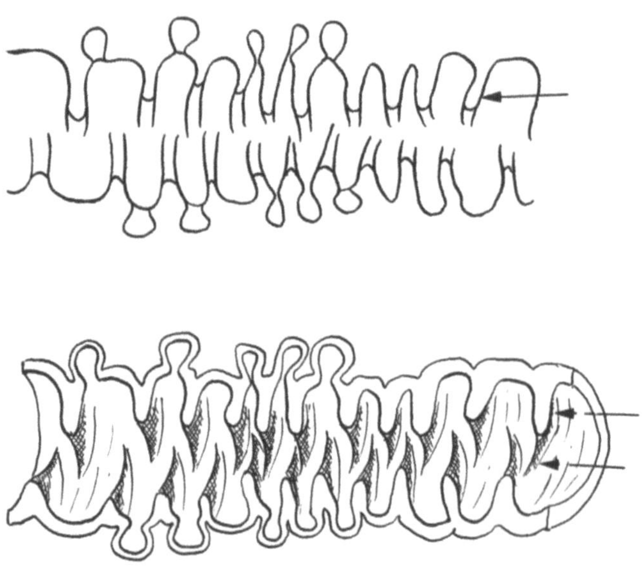

Fig. 8.4. Appearance of the colonic lumen corresponding to the radiologic zigzag or accordion image: **A,** radiologic zigzag or accordion aspect created by the bulging of colonic valves into the lumen *(arrow)*. **B,** longitudinal section of the same segment (sigmoid). The transverse folding is quite marked; the lumen is narrowed, which explains the image in **A**. The staggered configuration of the valves *(arrows)* is quite evident

8.2.2 Defects of the Colonic Muscular Coat

According to Morson [9], defects of the colonic muscular coat are the most striking aspects of sigmoid diverticular disease. There is a thickening and shortening of teniae associated with folding and diffuse or localized thickening of the circular muscle. Two appearances can be described for advanced sigmoid diverticulosis in segments opened following distension by formol solution. They correspond to classic radiologic descriptions detailed later in this chapter.

The first corresponds to the accordion or "zigzag" appearance ((Fig. 8.4). The colonic lumen appears transversely lined by highly projecting, compact semilunar folds. They are probably due to the accentuation of normal valves. They arise alternately from each of the mesenteric intertenial ridges and extend to the antimesenteric ridge, where they become effaced. These folds are staggered and delimit haustral cul-de-sacs, where diverticular openings originate. Histologically this infolding is due to corrugation of the mucosa and circular muscle where two layers are placed back to back (Fig. 8.5, A) or by localized thickening of the muscular coat (Fig. 8,5 C). The mucosa itself may fold, creating sharper finer corrugation (Fig. 8.5, B).

The second appearance corresponds to major diffuse thickening of the muscular coat. This narrows the caliber of the lumen, which is obstructed by mucous folds similar to jejunal folding (Fig. 8.5, d). Radiologically this corresponds to permanent spastic stenosis (muscular tumor).

8.2.3 Diverticular Inflammation

Diverticulitis refers to the inflammation of one or more diverticula as opposed to diverticulosis, which concerns only the presence of diverticula. This inflammation may remain localized in a diverticular pouch, but may spread by micro- or macroperforation and thus be the origin of a series of complications: localized or diffuse peritonitis, intramural dissecting abscess and pericolic abscesses with a possibility of fistula formation. Thus, the pathologic appearance of diverticulitis is well defined. The same is not true clinically or radiologically. Parks [12] emphasizes the lack of anatomic/clinical correlations. He notes that, according to Morson [8], one-third of the partial colectomies performed for diverticulitis showed no sign of inflammation and that an autopsy study by Hughes [6] showed 12% of subjects with diverticulosis as having had recent or long-standing diverticulitis and no suggestive clinical history. It is probable that very limited inflammation may go undetected clinically. On the other hand, it is certain that a diagnosis of diverticulitis is too often based on the discovery of nonspecific radiologic images. These are detailed later in this chapter.

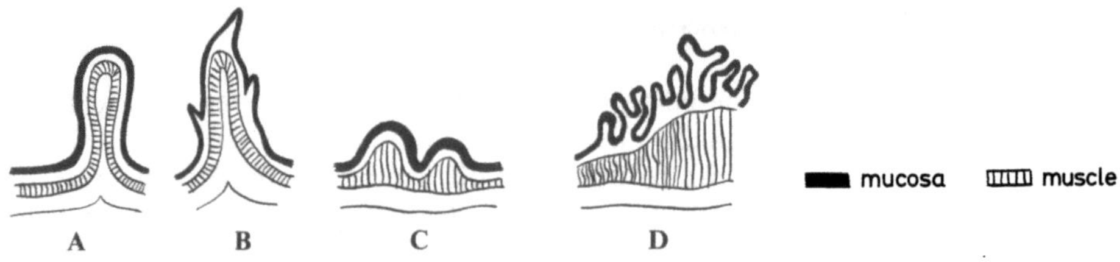

Fig. 8.5. Different types of muscular abnormalities identified in colonic diverticulosis: **A**, folding of the muscular coat; **B**, folding of the muscular coat with finer secondary folding of the mucosa; **C**, localized thickening of the circular muscle; **D**, diffuse thickening of the muscular coat with "jejunal" folding of the mucosa

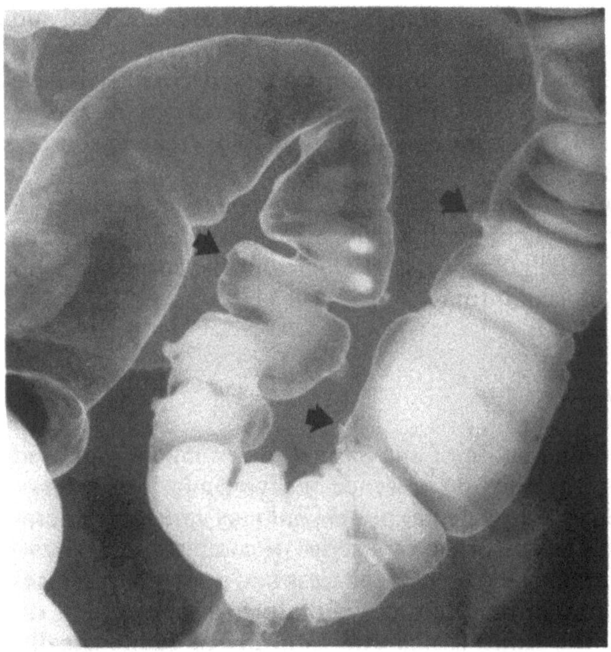

Fig. 8.6. Early sigmoid diverticulosis: immature diverticula are seen in profile *(arrows)*. More advanced diverticula and haustral alternation is also visible

8.3 Radiologic Aspects of Colonic Diverticulosis

The diagnosis of colonic diverticulosis is based on the radiologic examination.

8.3.1 Problems of Double Contrast in the Study of Diverticulosis

Contrary to what some still believe, colonic diverticulosis is not a contraindication to insufflation as long as it is performed gently. General rules of patient preparation are unchanged. The examination may be hindered by sigmoid hyperspasticity, which is frequent in this disease. In order to overcome this problem it is best to obtain radiographs of the sigmoid as early as possible in the examination (since distention of the sigmoid is best at this point) and to inject glucagon intravenously.

When an enema is indicated, care should be taken if a complication (diverticulitis, perforation) is suspected. In this case use of water-soluble single contrast enema is recommended. Double contrast enema should not be administered during acute attack. Preparation for these patients should be reduced or completely omitted.

8.3.2 Radiologic Features of Noncomplicated Diverticulosis

Radiologic signs include images of diverticula and associated caliber and haustral abnormalities.

8.3.2.1 Diverticular Images

According to Bockus [3], diverticulosis is more often detected by double contrast than by the standard technique. This is probably due to the facility with which diverticula can be demonstrated on the colonic walls (intermarginal aspect).

The immature diverticulum (Fig. 8.6) is seen in profile as a conical or triangular addition image several millimeters high. Frontally (where it is easily visible unlike in classic radiology), it is represented by an opaque spot when on the dependent surface and filled with barium (Fig. 8.7) and a ring shadow sometimes accompanied by a hat sign (formation of the image obeys the same rules as for a sessile polyp whose image is inversed) (Fig. 8.7).

The mature diverticulum has a characteristic appearance (Fig. 8.8): In profile we see a spherical addition image with clear regular borders joined to the wall by a fairly long, large neck. It varies in size from several millimeters to several centimeters. From a frontal or three-quarter view different images are possible: target, off-center target, ring shadow with a hat sign, or a dense rounded addition image with clear borders (if the diverticulum is filled with barium) (Fig. 8.9).

Its size and form may vary from one moment to the next, depending on the degree of colonic distension. The diverticulum may empty, changing from the appearance just described to one of a triangular bulge sometimes difficult to

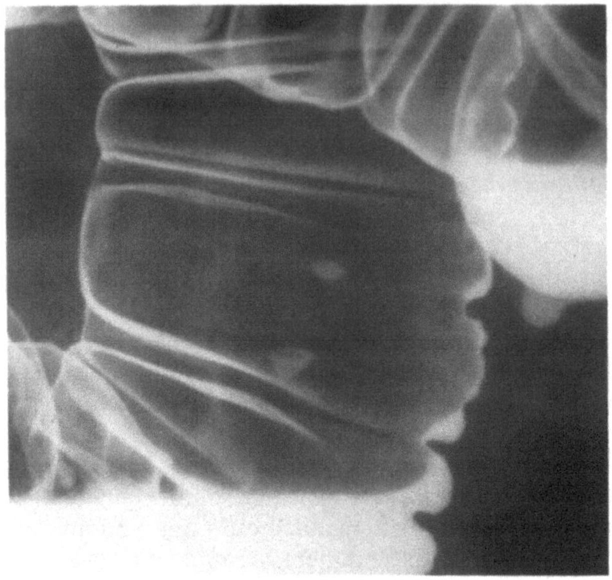

Fig. 8.7. Immature diverticula seen frontally in the intermarginal aspect. *Above,* opaque spot with clear borders. *Below,* ring shadow with hat sign. Diverticular necks are not yet present

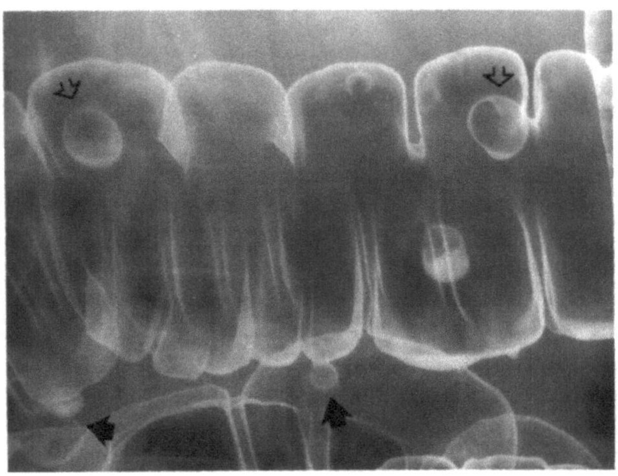

Fig. 8.8. Diverticula in the intermarginal aspect: target image, eccentric target image, with barium accumulation at the bottom *(open arrows)* (radiograph in upright position). Diverticula seen in profile on the margins *(black arrow)*

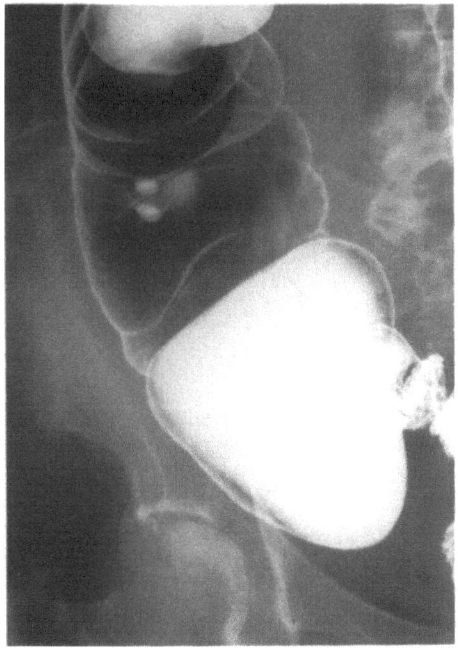

Fig. 8.9. Isolated diverticula in the right colon which appear as addition images with distinct borders with the patient in the prone position (they are located along the anterior antimesenteric tenia)

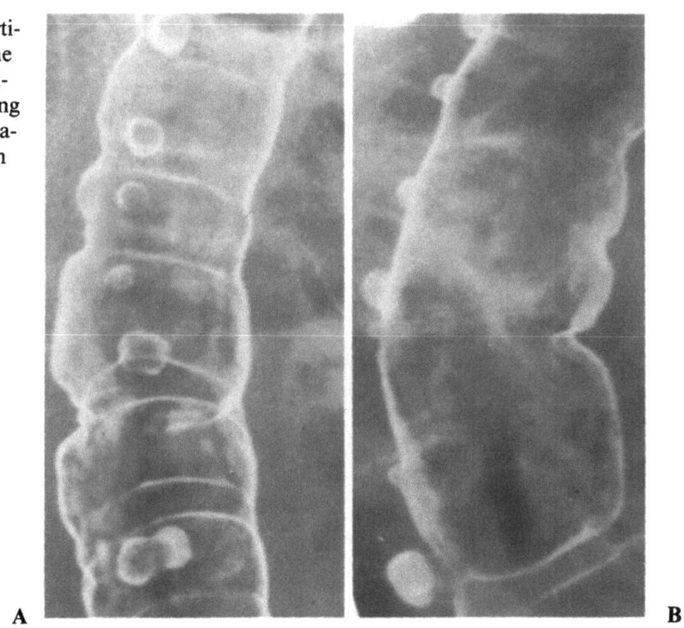

Fig. 8.10. Alignment of diverticula along the teniae. **A** In the descending colon, the diverticula are all seen frontally along the same tenia. **B** When the patient turns 90° they appear in profile

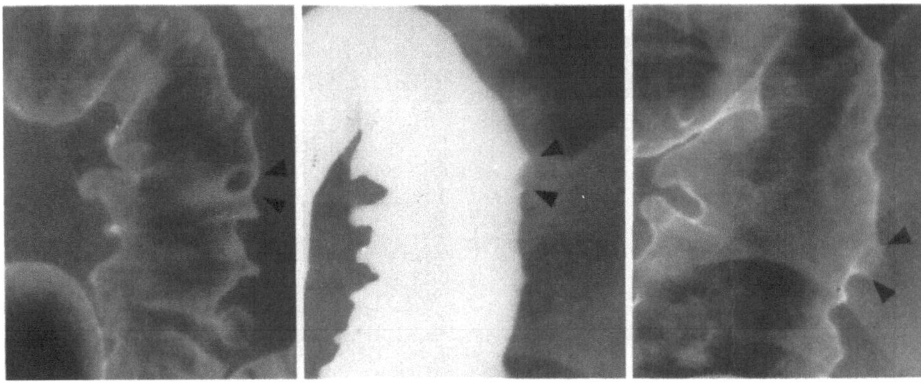

A, B, C

Fig. 8.11. Obstructed diverticulum: **A**, filling defect in the pool; **B**, filling defect partially situated in an addition image; **C**, ring shadow

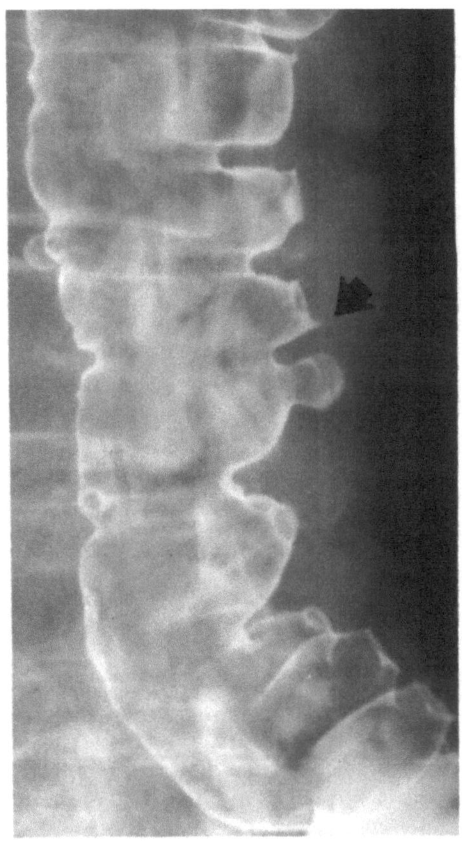

Fig. 8.12. Obstructed diverticula seen in profile. The tops of the haustrations are severed and appear straight or concave toward the exterior (characteristic calix image). They are often irregular and extended by a thread of barium *(arrow)* penetrating the diverticulum (spur image)

distinguish from the grooves separating mucous folds formed during colonic spasm. Actually, the images are seen at the top of the haustra (between the haustral clefts) or at the top of opaque grooves separating transversal folds of the mucosa (see Fig. 8.13). Their alignment along the teniae is quite apparent (Fig. 8.10).

Fecal residue may obstruct the diverticulum; its appearance changes: fecal matter in the diverticular pouch may cause the diverticular orifice to bulge into the colonic lumen. The resulting frontal image is either a ring shadow or a filling defect (Fig. 8.11). In profile, only the neck is visible. The top of the haustration is severed. If the obstruction is incomplete the presence of a fine thread of barium penetrating the diverticulum (spur image) which appears outside the colonic contour makes it possible to confirm the diagnosis (Fig. 8.12).

Diagnostic problems related to polyp images have already been discussed (see Chap. 3). Here, we will simply recall that a large-necked diverticulum may simulate a sessile polyp, a narrow-necked diverticulum may simulate a pedunculated or intermediate polyp, and an obstructed diverticulum may be simulated by a sessile polyp or adherent fecal matter. These problems only arise in cases of severe diverticulosis. Otherwise, obtaining the profile radiograph, using the pool sign, the image site (diverticula are rarely found in the rectum), the form variation, and the possible filling of diverticula make it possible to erase any doubt.

8.3.2.2 Caliber and Haustral Abnormalities

These are not always present and we can consider the following possibilities: (1) diverticulosis without haustral defects; (2) diverticulosis associated with discrete, nonspecific, even "physiologic" haustral defects that, when isolated, suggest a prediverticular state (alteration of haustra without diverticula); (3) diverticulosis with major haustral defects often misinterpreted as indicative of diverticulitis.

Diverticulosis May Not Be Accompanied by Caliber or Haustral Defects. This is usually the case with only one or a few diverticula. It is also characteristic of the localization the right colon. Haustral defects are much rarer here than in the descending colon.

Diverticulosis May Be Accompanied by Discreet, Nonspecific Caliber and Haustral Abnormalities. These abnormalities have been described in classic radiology but are also seen in double contrast despite the use of hypotonic medication. They are most often found in the left colon, especially in the sigmoid. They are represented by alternating haustrations: haustral clefts normally described as symmetric and facing one another in the sigmoid (actually they are rarely found here) are not seen face to face. Indentation occurs alternately from one border to the other, creating a staggered effect. They are shallow at this stage and delimit haustral cul-de-sacs. Diverticula originate at the top of these haustrations (Fig. 8.13).

They may also be represented by the palisade configuration, which appears to be due to an increase in transverse folding sometimes predominant in the antimesenteric ridge (Fig. 8.14).

Significance of Discreet Haustral Defects. In our opinion only those images

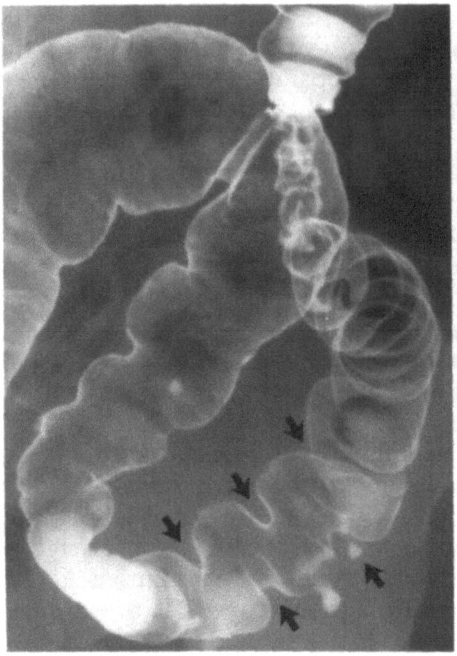

8.13

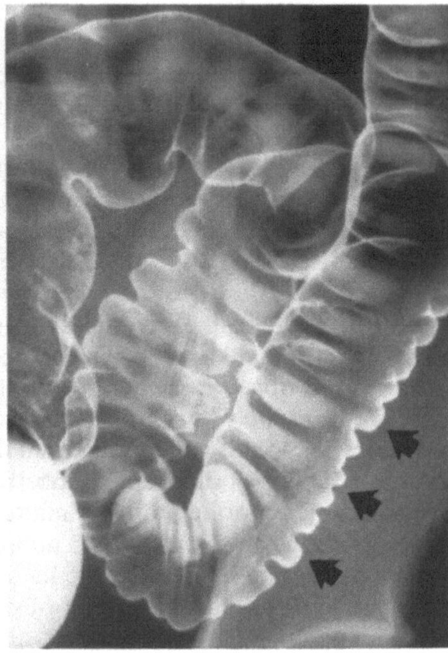

8.14

Fig. 8.13. Alternating haustrations in the sigmoid *(arrows)*. Note the spasticity of the descending colon

Fig. 8.14. Unilateral palisade configuration *(arrows)*

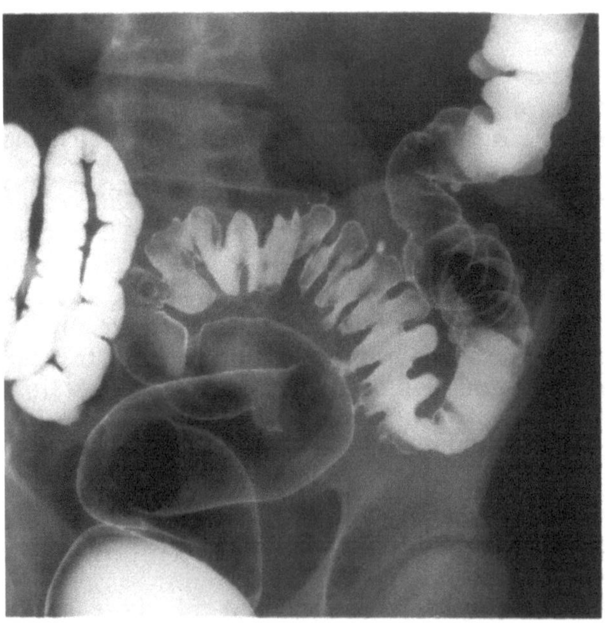

Fig. 8.15. Characteristic zigzag appearance (noncomplicated diverticulosis). The position of the diverticula at the top of the haustral cul-de-sacs is clearly visible

which persist in a sufficiently insufflated colon, should be taken into consideration. Similar transitory images may appear in normal subjects during filling. The significance of these discreet persistent defects is unclear. They are found in association with, as well as in the absence of, diverticula. In this case we speak of "irritable colon" and of "prediverticular" state. Williams [14] has experimentally reproduced these defects in the cadaver by shortening the teniae. They may thus reflect a state of colonic hypertonia with transitory or definitive muscular defects where tenia contraction plays a major role. The pathologic nature of these haustral distortions has not yet been confirmed.

Diverticulosis May Be Accompanied by Major Haustral Defects. Two images may form: the "zigzag" and spastic stenosis. These images have for a long time been misinterpreted as representative of the inflammatory lesions of diverticulitis. We now know they only represent advanced anatomic and dynamic changes which can be present in the absence of all diverticular inflammation. The "zigzag" (Fig. 8.15) or accordion (Fig. 8.16) images are due to alternated, highly compact, deep and uniform haustrations which separate the haustral cul-de-sacs. The "spastic" stenosis image represents a narrowing, usually over several centimeters, which progressively brings upper and lower segments together. When analyzable the mucous folding of this affected area has been shown to be conserved (Fig. 8.17).

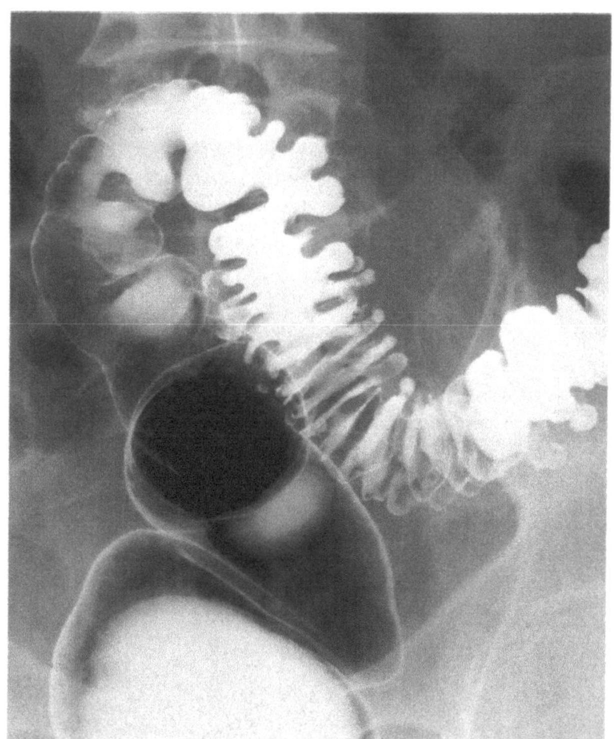

Fig. 8.16. Accordion image: the folding is denser than in the previous radiographs

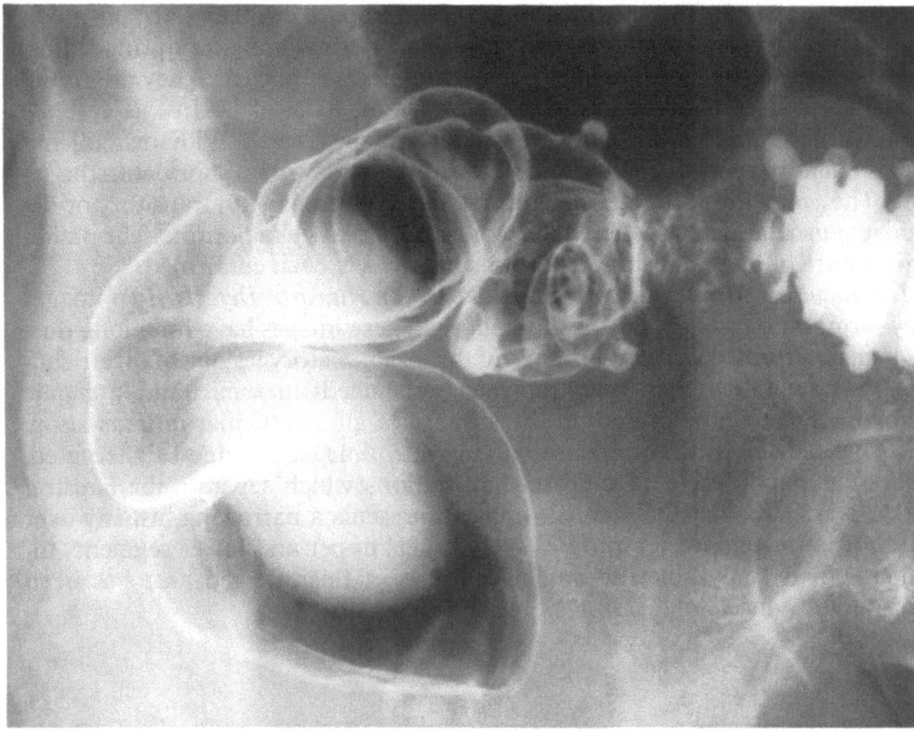

Fig. 8.17. Spastic stenosis in sigmoid diverticulosis. This image in itself is not sufficient to confirm the diverticulitis. Here the clinical findings are essential

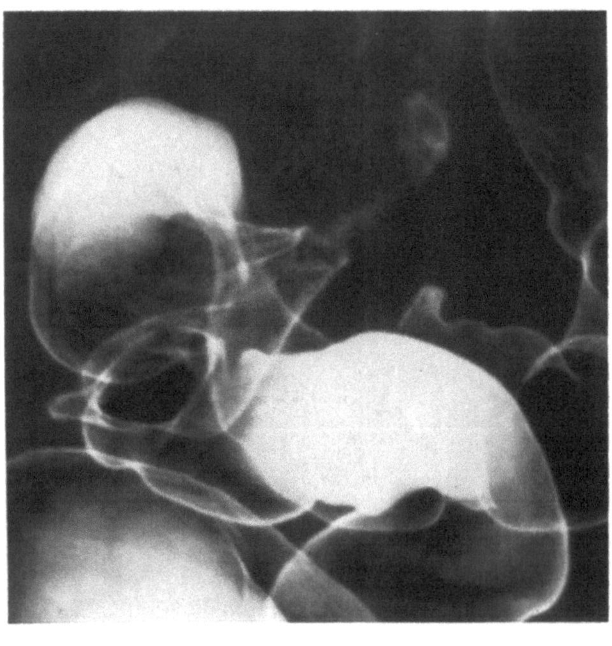

Fig. 8.18. Minimal escape in sigmoid diverticulitis (acute regressive episode unrecognized 1 month earlier). The examination was well tolerated without complication. Note the absence of peridiverticular retraction

8.4 Diverticulosis and Diverticulitis

Often, a diagnosis of "diverticulitis" is incorrectly reached based on radiologic evidence. The images we have just described (major haustral defects and spastic stenosis images) are still too often considered as representing inflammatory lesions, whereas they only indicate muscular defects due to diverticulosis. Two essential points must be emphasized:

1. Haustral defects, which may be considerable, can be present in the absence of all inflammation.
2. Diverticulitis may not be accompanied by any haustral defect.

Since the first stage of diverticulitis is inflammation of the diverticular pouch [5], distortion of one or several diverticula by a small abscess and their nonopacification by the barium were considered to be early signs of diverticulitis [16]. In that such images are also found for simple diverticulosis without infection, due to fecal residue, they are only of minor value in diagnosing diverticulitis. The diagnosis of diverticulitis by barium enema must only be based on reliable signs: this diagnosis can be confirmed when the presence of colonic diverticula is associated with one of the following signs:

1. Barium escape or extraluminal air (Fig. 8.18).
2. Extrinsic compression of the colon by an abscess (Fig. 8.19)
3. Presence of a dissecting abscess. In the sigmoid region, this type of abscess usually appears as a track several centimeters long parallel to the colonic wall. This together with the original lumen forms the double-track sign [4].

In addition to these signs the radiological discovery of diverticulosis (association of diverticula and haustral and caliber abnormalities) in conjunction with a probable clinical picture suffices to diagnose a case of diverticulitis. Other radiologic techniques can be used to demonstrate the abscess: ultrasound, computed tomography and gallium 67 scintigraphy.

Some cases of diverticulitis may be first discovered by the radiologic examination (Fig. 8.18). In general, this occurs for patients whose clinical symptoms are misleading. In all the cases we observed, barium leakage was never a problem, since the infection is often well "contained" and barium escape quite limited.

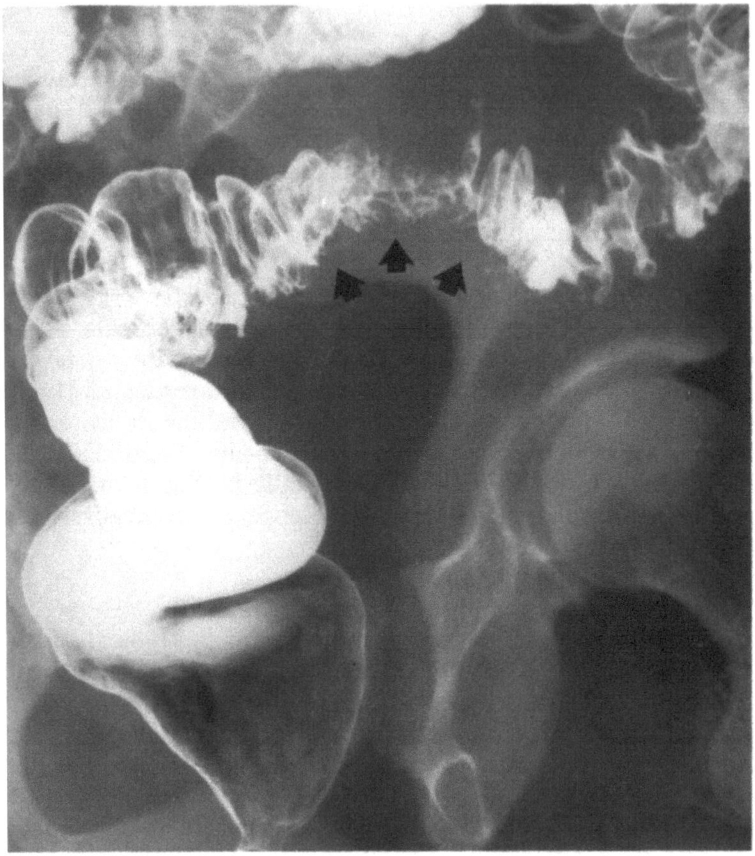

Fig. 8.19. Perisigmoid abscess: stenosis with conservation of mucous folding; progressive joining of adjacent segments; compression of the inferior margin of the sigmoid makes it possible to confirm the diverticulitis

8.5 Diverticulosis and Associated Lesions

The last step in the double contrast examination of diverticulosis is the search for associated lesions. Diverticulosis, polyps, and cancer all affect the same age group. The association of polyps or colonic carcinoma and diverticulosis creates two problems: recognizing a polyp and differentiating between spastic and neoplastic stenosis.

8.5.1 The Detection of Associated Polyps Requires

A high-quality examination and a thorough, detailed interpretation. Particular attention should be given to the search for: filling defects, especially if large or polycyclic; the longitudinal image of a stalk across the haustra; and a target image on a valvular fold (diverticula are not found on valves). A large number of diverticula may make this search difficult and necessitate a colonoscopic examination.

8.5.2 Differentiation Between the Colonic Stenosis Caused by Cancer and That Caused by Diverticulosis

Classic signs favoring the spastic (or inflammatory) nature of colonic stenosis are: (1) the progressive transition between normal and pathologic segments (absence of the tumoral pole is clear with double contrast), (2) the length of the stenosis (often as much as several centimeters), (3) the conservation of mucous folding within the stenosis and the absence of tumoral ulceration, and (4) the variation between successive examinations. These elements are clearly detected by double contrast; however, the radiologic examination cannot always establish a formal diagnosis [2].

8.6 Conclusion

The clinical symptoms aside, double contrast provides for a thorough study of colonic diverticulosis. All classic aspects of colonic tonus abnormalities can be demonstrated and a positive diagnosis is reached more often than with the standard technique. Diagnosis of associated lesions poses no real problem other than that of polyp detection when diverticula are numerous.

References

1. Arfwidsson S (1964) Pathogenesis of multiple diverticula of the sigmoid colon in diverticular disease. Acta Chirurgica Scandinava (Suppl) 342
2. Bertrand J (1972) La diverticulose colique. Expansion Scientifique Française
3. Bockus (1974) Gastroenterology, T II Saunders, Philadelphia pp 973-996
4. Ferruci JT, Ragsdale BD, Barett P, Vickery AL, Dreyfus JR (1976) Double tracking in the sigmoïd colon. Radiology 120: 307-312
5. Fleischner FG, Si-Chun Ming, Henken EM (1964) Revised concepts on diverticular disease of the colon. Radiology 83: 859-871
6. Hughes LE (1969) Post mortem survey of diverticular disease. Gut 10: 336-351
7. Meyers MA, Volberg F, Katzen B, Alonso D, Abbot G (1973) The angioarchitecture of colonic diverticula. Radiology 108: 249-261
8. Morson BC (1975) Pathology of diverticular disease of the colon. Clinics Gastroenterol 4: 37-52
9. Morson BC (1963) The muscle abnormality in diverticular disease of the sigmoid colon. Brit J Radiol 36: 385-392
10. Painter NS, Burkitt DP (1975) Diverticular disease of the colon: a 20th century problem. Clinics Gastroenterol 4: 3-21
11. Painter NS, Truelove SC, Ardran GM, Tuckey M (1965) Segmentation and the localization of intra luminal pressures in the human colon, with special reference to the pathogenesis of colonic diverticula. Gastroenterology 49: 169-177
12. Parks TC (1975) Natural history of diverticular disease of the colon. Clinics Gastroenterol 4: 53-69
13. Taylor I, Duthie HL (1976) Bran tablets and diverticular disease. Br Med J 1: 988-990
14. Williams J (1963) Changing emphasis in diverticular disease of the colon. Brit J Radiol 36: 393-406
15. Williams J (1967) Diverticular disease of the colon without diverticula. Radiology 98: 401-412
16. Williams I, Schnyder P (1983) Diverticula in Alimentary Tract Radiology. 3rd edn. p 1690-1112. Mosby, St. Louis pp 1690-1712

9 Conclusion

The double contrast technique represents a considerable advance among the various methods of colonic examination. Our 10 years of experience using double contrast have shown it to be a relatively easy procedure, providing certain prerequisistes are fulfilled.

These include willingness to use double contrast and to obtain high-quality examinations, all of which requires some effort on the part of the radiologist. Certain technical conditions are essential: reserving a specific area in the hospital for the patient's preparation, personnel cooperation in light of the new procedures used, and learning the technique from experienced radiologists. Also important is the need for the radiologist to obtain the correct patient preparation by formulating his prescriptions according to the clinical picture. Finally, the examination itself must comply with very strict quality standards and its thorough interpretation calls for new rules, which must be acquired.

When these prerequisites are achieved, double contrast becomes a very satisfying examination for the radiologist, due to the wealth of information it provides. Its main advantage is the possibility of early detection and thus efficient treatment of rectocolic cancer.

MIX
Papier aus verantwortungsvollen Quellen
Paper from responsible sources
FSC® C105338

If you have any concerns about our products,
you can contact us on
ProductSafety@springernature.com

In case Publisher is established outside the EU,
the EU authorized representative is:
Springer Nature Customer Service Center GmbH
Europaplatz 3, 69115 Heidelberg, Germany

Printed by Libri Plureos GmbH
in Hamburg, Germany